INSTANT ANSWERS 4 HEALTHY KIDS

❖

Acknowledgments

I want to extend my deepest gratitude to Demis Giamalis for the front cover design and Clayton Pearson for going beyond the second mile in assisting me through the whole creative process; the finished sleeve and release of this book. Many thanks go to Walton Mendelson for the final touches and to my children and grandchildren. And for the little acts of service: you're a champion Shane. I couldn't have done this without you!

Thank you all so much!

Instant Answers 4 Healthy Kids

Cheryl Gi

www.answers4healthykids.com

Legal Notice

While every attempt has been made to verify information provided in this publication, Help 4 Healthy Kids, does not assume any responsibility for errors, omissions, or contrary interpretation of the subject matter herein.

This publication is not intended to replace advice or treatment from health professionals. Help 4 Healthy Kids wishes to stress that the information contained herein may be subject to varying country laws and regulations. All users are encouraged to expand their knowledge through competent health professionals and further research as required.

The purchaser or reader of this publication assumes responsibility for how they perceive and use this information. The author assumes no responsibility or liability whatsoever on the behalf of any purchaser or reader of this material.

Any perceived slights of specific individuals or organizations are unintentional.

Typsetting: Help 4 Healthy Kids
Cover Graphics: Help 4 Healthy Kids
Printing: www.CreateSpace.com, USA

To purchase additional copies of this material or request permission, please contact us at
info@help4healthykids.com

Thank you for purchasing Instant Answers 4 Healthy Kids

Preface

This book will become your best friend. It was created to help you overcome sickness instead of having sickness overcome you. It will help give you back those nights of blissful sleep and days free of the anxiety associated with caring for sick children. This book will also give you insight into improving *your own* health.

It may come as a surprise to you, as you discover how your infant/child can avoid the misery associated with various stages of development, like teething or ears, nose and throat infections, plus many more. You will be amazed as you witness an often rapid recovery at any age, by simply giving your child the tools his/her body needs to fight back. Along the way, this manual will become not just a learning curve for you and your family, but a close companion and invaluable resource.

By studying the impact of vitamins, and applying what I've learned with my family, myself and others, I have reduced my visits to the doctor by more than 40% over the past 30 plus years and I've saved a great deal on medical expenses. I am a living 30 year case study and a testimony of applied/remedial nutrition that has never failed. I saved my children the suffering that comes with ill health, and avoided the anguish associated with it. I am indebted to the pioneer efforts of Adelle Davis* whose knowledge in nutrition has delivered such amazing success. This document is not directed at academics, but more for women who want straight answers. For this reason I've taken some liberties with formal writing protocol and used my 'speaking to you face to face' style. The content of this book has been condensed to essential knowledge to set you on the path to good health and in a way that is easy to follow. It covers key information on the role and impact of vitamins and alerts you to the chief contributors of ill health that the majority of people are unaware of; so that preventive and curative action can be taken.

_____

* All the case studies presented here outside of my own, come from 'Let's Have Healthy Children' and 'Let's Get Well' (now out of print) by Adelle Davis: Davis attended Purdue University from 1923 to 1925 and received her Bachelor of Arts degree from the University of California at Berkeley in 1927. After dietetic training at Bellevue and Fordham Hospitals in New York, she became supervisor of nutrition for Yonkers Public Schools from 1928 through 1930. From 1931 through 1938, Davis was a consulting nutritionist in Oakland and Los Angeles, California, did postgraduate work at Columbia University and the University of California at Los Angeles, and received her Master of Science degree in Biochemistry from the University of Southern California

Cheryl Gi

My philosophy is this: "If it gets results then it works.... If it works then it is worth pursuing."

THIS ... is worth pursuing.

CONTENTS

CHAPTER 1: VITAMINS EXPLAINED: WHY WE NEED THEM . . . **11**

CHAPTER 2: MY STORY: HOW IT ALL BEGAN **20**

CHAPTER 3: ANSWERS WHEN YOU NEED THEM A – A **28**

CHAPTER 4: ANSWERS WHEN YOU NEED THEM B – C **46**

CHAPTER 5: ANSWERS WHEN YOU NEED THEM D –V **62**

CHAPTER 6: SUPPLEMENTS DURING PREGNANCY **83**

CHAPTER 7: WHAT TO DO WHEN THINGS GO WRONG **93**

CHAPTER 8: TWO AMAZING VITAMINS **108**

CHAPTER 9: CAUSE AND EFFECT vs VITAMINS **116**

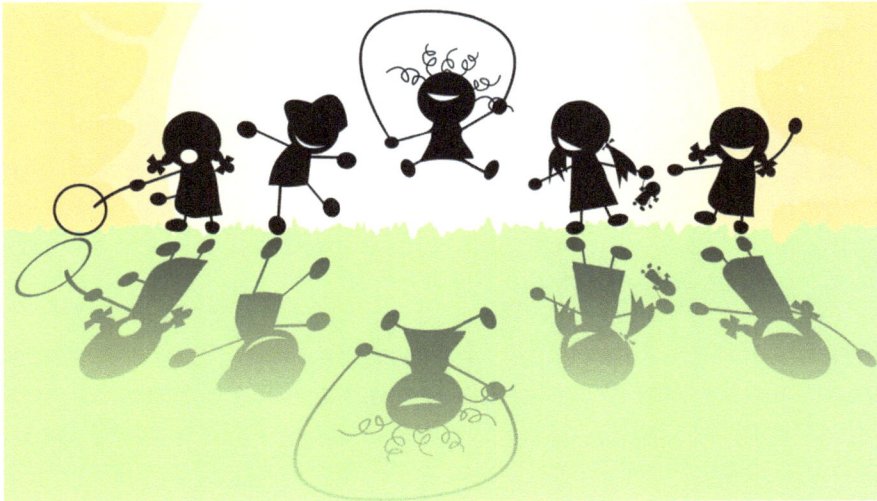

Chapter 1 – VITAMINS EXPLAINED: WHY WE NEED THEM

Whether we are aware of it or not, whether we believe it or not, our bodies need a certain quota of nutrients every day in order to function at an optimal level. Our body is designed to function in a specific way. It has built in mechanisms to prevent illness and disease, to fight and overcome illness and to repair and maintain itself. Our body's ability to carry out these functions varies according to the tools or nutrients we give it. Inherited deficiencies and nutrient intake during pregnancy have an impact on the health of children. It follows that what we put into our body is of paramount importance.

We often hear the term 'a balanced diet' thrown at us. But is there such a thing? Perhaps a century ago there might have been, but not any more. As society has 'advanced', things have gone a little awry. Life has become fast paced. Everything has to be 'instant' or time saving because time is in short supply and time is money. So we have an abundance of processed foods and fast food outlets available. Supermarkets have a lot to answer for, as they purchase fruit and vegetables **before** they are fully ripe, so that the produce keeps better on their shelves. This reduces the nutrient value, simply because fruit and vegetables need to ripen fully to develop their full nutrient potential. Or the opposite occurs, where fruit is kept in cold storage for months. Just how old **is** it when we buy it?

*Picking fruit and vegetables **early,** robs them (and us) of vitamins that are vital to our well-being.* I have come across a number of articles that support this very issue. One article I found in a magazine that is released by a Pharmacy chain in Australia, stated that a discovery was made that tomatoes now have about a third of their appointed nutrient value.

I immediately thought, 'As if Mother Nature is going to target only tomatoes!' Of course not! Over time, the soil that **ALL** plants grow in is being leeched of nutrients—so **ALL** plants are affected. As a result, we get short changed without being aware of it. It comes as no surprise then that as this has been happening silently for decades, illness and disease has been growing.

As consumers, we have innocently and naively assumed that the produce we buy is okay. I am here to tell you it is NOT. Yes, it is edible generally, but we deceive ourselves if we think it is providing a balanced diet or adequate nutrients. Our best option is to buy 'organic' grown produce. Although the measure of 'organic' can be a little nebulous, there are organizations that demand specific standards in order for a grower to have their product/s 'certified organic' stamp of approval. A grower could apply a few kilos of fertilizer for example, or 1 ton of fertilizer and still label it 'organic'. In Australia, the ACO (Australian Certified Organic), has a key role in this process. Consumers need to look for suppliers of certified organic fruit, vegetables, meat and poultry. Regardless, 'certified organic' is still the better option. Or you could grow your own fruit and vegetables.

Another issue impacting our health is pollution / toxic levels. Since World War II, when certain metals and resources became scarce, manufacturers were forced to develop alternatives. As a result we have plastics, metal alloys and all kinds of synthetic resources available today. We bought these products and they continued to be produced without giving too much thought about the impact on our health or environment. Pollution is everywhere – no one can escape it. It is in the water that we wash in and consume each day. It is in our oceans killing the kelp and contaminating the fish that we eat. It's in the soil where we grow fruit and vegetables. Instead of nutrient rich soil, we have pollutant rich soil that is nutrient poor.

Collectively, there are countless toxins that have been released— into the air we breathe, the soil, the water, the houses we live in, and the cars we drive. These are issues that we have little control over. And it doesn't end there. I was horrified to discover the degree of toxins found present in infant blood tests and revealed in the excerpts that follow.

"The report, Body Burden—The Pollution in Newborns, by the Washington, D.C.-based Environmental Working Group, detected 287 chemicals in the umbilical cord blood of 10 newborns. Of those chemicals, 76 cause cancers in humans or animals, 94 are toxic to the brain and nervous system and 79 cause birth defects or abnormal development in animal tests."

"What's most startling is that we have such a wide range of compounds in us the moment we are born," said Tim Kropp, senior toxicologist for the project. "Babies don't use any consumer products, they don't work in a factory and yet they're already starting off with a load of these chemicals."

"In a benchmark study released today, researchers found an average of 200 industrial compounds, pollutants and other chemicals in the umbilical cord blood of newborns, including

*seven dangerous pesticides some banned in the United States
more than 30 years ago."*

It is not my intention to alarm you, but this is scary stuff! We
can't ignore it any longer and we certainly can't wait around for
politicians to get their act together. They have their own agenda.
Considering the political posturing, subterfuge and deceipt politicians can generate, it begs the question: 'Do they really want
to?' They are too busy manipulating the economy and pander-
ing to the corporations that help fund their election campaigns
that keep them in power. Let's not hold our breath waiting for
them to make the first move. The longer we procrastinate the
greater the risk to our family's health. There are things **we** can
do and this book is a part of that process.

Every time you use personal care products, when you bath your
baby, have a shower, wash your hands or hair, clean your teeth,
and the list goes on, *you put toxins into your body. These are
transferred to your unborn baby. Every time we heat up food in
the microwave using a plastic container or plastic wrap, we release dioxin in to the food and increase our risk of cancer when
we eat it. Please, if you must use a microwave, use glass or
ceramic containers to avoid this.*

According to Dr Samuel Epstein of the Cancer Prevention Coalition, from conception (inside our mother's womb) until our life
ends, we continue to take toxins into our body. Is it any wonder
that adults and children are getting sick? One in three people
(now closer to I in every 2), including children are suffering with
cancer, and the statistics are increasing. Allergies and Diabetes
have become common in society. Disease is on the rise at an
alarming rate.

Our bodies are being saturated with toxins; to such an extent
that <u>we can't escape them</u> and **more importantly, our bodies
cannot cope with them.** We need to take action to combat it.
Combat is the perfect word here. We can no longer take our
health for granted and we cannot reverse our polluted environ-

ment overnight. Nor can we continue to place the entire responsibility of our health in the hands of pharmaceutical companies and our failing health system.

What we **can** do is look after ourselves and take action. No one else will. It took me half a lifetime to learn that we can't change other people. We can only change ourselves or remove ourselves from the problem. Unfortunately there is no where to go, to 'remove ourselves' from this situation.

That means accepting responsibility for it ourselves. It means taking back a measure of control, of the health of our families. If I can do it, so can you.

TIP NUMBER ONE: BE ALERT

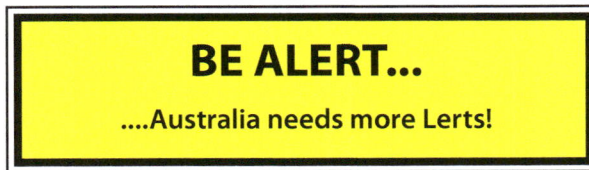

> # BE ALERT...
> ....Australia needs more Lerts!

*I couldn't resist sharing this yellow car sticker. From a distance all I could read was, 'BE ALERT,' and thought it might be something profound. When I drove closer and read the small print I cracked up laughing. We **do** need to be alert!*

I have in my possession a book called, "Unreasonable Risk" by Dr. Samuel Epstein MD and Chairman of the Cancer Prevention Coalition (U.S.)—a real eye opener. Dr. Epstein has a booklet that gives a list of some of the safe alternative products on the market and recommends only one company's products (Neways), which he personally tested and has certified them safe. All the other manufacturers he approached would not let him in the door. (I wonder why). There are other companies that produce safe products, but they are as rare as hen's teeth. Personally, I started out with, Neways and then discovered a few individual 'safe' products along the way that I intersperse with these.

If you can find any personal care product on supermarket shelves that does not contain Sodium Laurel Sulphate (in various forms) or Propylene Glycol, I would have to see it to believe it. House cleaning products are no better. I have checked the super market products in question, and after considerable time found it to be an exercise in futility. Checking contents has become a constant practice when shopping at supermarkets etc. You may find an exception in the health and vitamin sections, but even some of these are contaminated. These two chemicals alone are carcinogens. Carcinogens contribute to Cancer. Do you want to keep allowing these toxins into the bodies of your children? The skin is the largest organ of the body and whatever goes on the skin, finds its way to the blood stream.

What I have previously discussed is just the tip of the iceberg, but I believe you are beginning to get the picture. If you do a 'Google' search for "an updated list of carcinogens," you will get 8 pages of them, and information on how they impact on the body. It would be ludicrous to go through 8 pages of carcinogens each time we went to the supermarket. However, Sodium Laurel Sulphate, Propylene Glycol and any 'parabens' or chemical with the word 'propyl' in it, are dangerous. These are found in products we use every day. Invest in a magnifying glass to read the contents though.

Check and avoid food dyes, additives and preservatives too.

Manufacturers take advantage of our ignorance and inertia. Instead of printing the actual name of a preservative or additive, they print the number that represents it—knowing full well that most people can't be bothered checking out what it is. Please, don't walk around with 'tunneled vision'—the price is too high.

Without the toxins, we need to take vitamin supplements to replace what is missing in our food. *With the toxins,* the threat of disease and degree of risk is so high that we have no choice but to take action.

While the body is trying to cope with the toxins, *it uses its existing resources* to do so—resources that are urgently needed in other parts of the body to maintain it. **These same toxins reduce the body's ability to absorb what meager nutrients we have, creating a climate that *invites* disease.** As toxins have been discovered in new born infants (page13) we need to get our head around these issues. We need to understand and take action.

From everyone's perspective, irrespective of age:
- We need to avoid using contaminated products and find safe alternatives.
- We need to take powerful anti-oxidants to help get existing toxins out of our system. Or a detox treatment.
- We need to drink huge amounts of water to help flush out the toxins. Water *without* Fluoride.
- We need to take high-potency vitamins and minerals just "to keep on keeping on" and meet our bodies' needs.
- For infants/toddlers these actions combined will provide the tools to fight back:
- The safest anti oxidants for infants are found in fruit juices, e.g. blue berries, red grapes, cherries, apples, pomegranates.
- Studies have shown that breast milk provides better anti oxidant effectiveness than formula.

Please remember that recovery takes time and each individual has a different set of variables to deal with. With practice you will become more in tune with how your body responds and how your children respond. What a joy it will be to see your children emerge into a healthier, happier existence.

Drawing from my experience, I have found the following to be evident:

Not enough nutrients present or no supplements taken...
- Poor to no protection.

- Inability to function on an acceptable, healthy level.
- Significant vulnerability to any illness/disease
- Having to suffer those illnesses—sometimes causing damage that can impact your health in the future.
- Discomfort and suffering for the victim. Anguish and stress for the caregiver.

Barely adequate intake of vitamins/nutrients =
- Some protection (as opposed to none) from illness.
- The level of 'satisfactory health' fluctuates according to the level of nutrients.
- Vulnerability to illness.
- Having to suffer some illness which may have been avoided.
- Suffering and inconvenience for the victim. Some stress/ distress for the caregiver.

Ideal/high intake of vitamins/nutrients =
- Excellent protection against viral, bacterial, fungal and other infections.
- Ability to function at optimal level i.e. an individual's personal best.
- Vulnerability to sickness is not an issue / extremely rare.
- Any illness is minimized and recovery is faster.
- Sickness and discomfort is rare, mild and manageable. Caregiver can relax.

Simply put: when you become sick with *anything* from a cold to serious health conditions, it is a clear indication that the body is in distress and needs help.

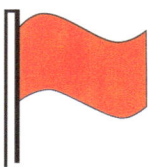

Sickness of any kind or measure is a red flag telling you the body is lacking in basic nutrients (vitamins/ minerals/water, etc) and cannot protect, function or overcome the illness—until it is given the nutrients it needs.

Sickness is the body's distress signal for more weapons (nutrients) to fight disease and achieve optimal health.

Medication/drugs on the other hand, have a tendency to treat the symptoms while ignoring the root cause of the problem.

This does people and children a huge *dis*service. *It masks the true nature of the illness*, fools us into thinking that we are well—because the symptoms have gone—when in fact the *cause* of the illness is STILL THERE.

Think about that. This leaves the body in a more vulnerable and degenerative state, to struggle on its own.

We really need to start nourishing and protecting our bodies and our children's, from the inside out, with the knowledge to do so.

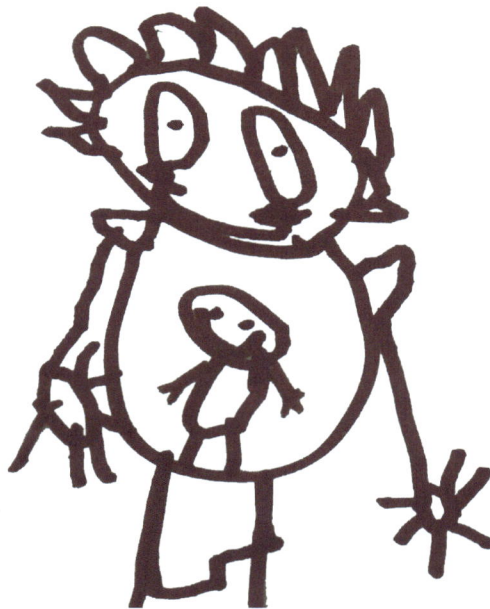

"I love you Mum and Dad 0000 XXXX"

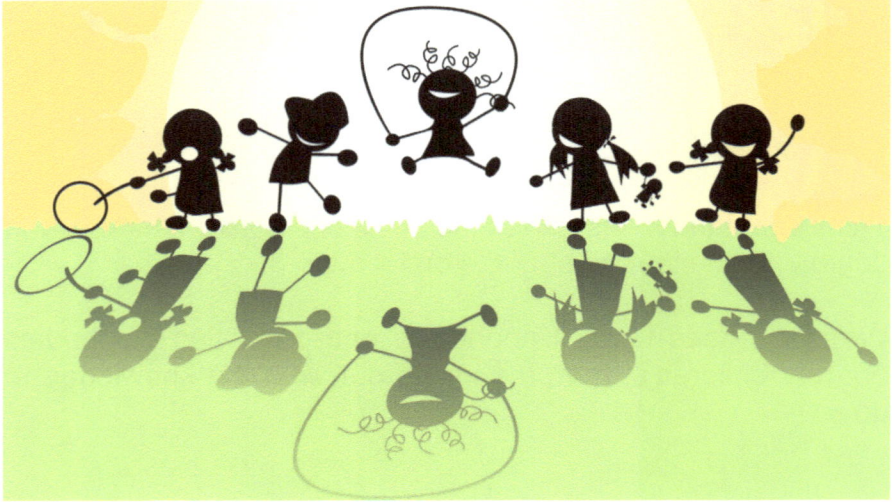

Chapter 2 – MY STORY: HOW IT ALL BEGAN

In 1976 I was reclining in a hospital bed, 4 months pregnant with my first baby, having arrived by ambulance with serious pain in my kidneys. I was distressed. All sorts of tests were done. The pain eventually subsided but the tests revealed nothing to explain its presence—no infection, nothing. They decided that it must have been something to do with the position of the baby.

Well I have to say that I didn't buy that idea. It had been the exact same pain I had experienced during a kidney infection in the past. After tests and a few days of observation, I was sent home. However, I had to continue my prenatal checkups with the Head of Obstetrics; Dr. Eileen Connon. Dr. Connon had shown me a graph of the baby's growth rate and pointed out that the baby was under-sized. She added that if the baby's size did not reach desired levels, I would have to stay in the hospital. That idea did not appeal to me at all. There was no way I was going to let that happen.

My immediate response was to go to the health shop, where I found a book by an American Nutritionist, Adelle Davis. I started reading and I couldn't put the book down. In fact I devoured it. From that day forward. I never looked back. That book became my 'bible' and *after 6 weeks of applying the advice contained in it, the growth rate of the baby shot up to 'normal.'* After explaining to Dr. Connon how I achieved this she said, "Yes, it's an excellent book." I nearly fell off the chair or in this case the bed. She had not only read the book but approved of my actions. Wow!

What I've learned in the years that followed has been invaluable. My source of information has never failed me in thirty years. Never. I took all the supplements recommended diligently. All through pregnancy, breast feeding and prior to pregnancy with my other children. During times of stress, like teething for example, I gave my children anti-stress vitamins as advised and they never experienced the traumas associated with teething. There was no misery, crying, sleepless nights, 'runny nose' or "because she's teething" to deal with. I learned how to deal with jaundice, colic, and a host of other conditions associated with infants and children.

When I was pregnant with my third child, my doctor, Dr. John Svigos said to me, "I don't have to worry about you Cheryl, you're always so healthy." That was music to my ears, but he didn't realize the vigilance involved on my part. It was not always like that though. I was not a particularly healthy child growing up. I had the usual childhood diseases like mumps and measles, and caught just about anything that was going around.

I grew up in the country and In spite of the more wholesome foods I was raised on, I continued to suffer respiratory tract infections, even though my tonsils had been removed as a toddler. The fast food industry wasn't available. We had home-grown vegetables, our own chickens, fresh fish that my father caught milk straight from the cow and the list goes on. It is clear to me *now*; that my body was *not* getting the quantity of nutrients it needed back then. But that was when I had no knowledge of such things. Now I know better.

The question is: Why let children suffer with ill health, when there are ways of avoiding that suffering?"

It continues to trouble me, why so many children are 'allowed' to suffer with certain conditions because parents are continually told, and led to believe, that it's 'normal'. And hey, I've been sucked into that state too. But how does that make it alright? Why do we accept so many *unhealthy* conditions and shrug them off as 'normal?' If half the population decided to go out and steal, would that make stealing 'okay' or 'normal?' If the other half of the population decided to swing from trees and make monkey noises, would everyone just shrug and say 'Darwin was right!' and accept the weird behavior? Do you see what I am saying? It is always good to do your own research, and then you have something to compare it with and can make an informed decision. By all means, search for more information. This book is not the be all and end all of nutritional remedies, but it's a good beginning.

It is also a good practice to measure 'normal' by the yardstick of optimal health, NOT by the number of children who get sick with the same condition. It's a little like the 'dumbing down' process in schools. The standards are lowered so that young Tommy can pass even though he has not grasped the knowledge well enough to handle the next level of learning. Even when this is done under the guise of social development, it is a 'Band-Aid' action, covering but not addressing the real problem. Where your children (and yourself) are concerned, I urge you not to accept anything less than the best level of health and education.

I have the greatest respect for the medical profession but they don't know *everything and like all human beings they make mistakes.* You need to question things. At the risk of repeating myself, you need to arm yourself with information so that you can ask intelligent questions and get intelligent answers from a cross section of health professionals. If you don't get satisfactory answers or results then seek alternatives. And don't stop until you find the solutions—or until you find something that works for you.

I have encountered a number of health professionals over my life time, that have made a statement or a diagnosis based on mistaken information or ignorance. And it isn't their fault that some things are missing from their training. I've lost count of the times I've heard the medical profession say there is 'no known cure' or they don't know what causes a particular malady, but hand you a 'here take this' medication. I've found medical web-sites, books and magazines telling me the same things. There are doctors who still don't know what causes colic, or what causes chronic fatigue, for example; but documented evidence has been available for 2 to 3 decades to enlighten them. Unfortunately, these two examples are not alone.

Because it is outside the realm of their knowledge, these experts have made errors of judgment in many cases, resulting in misdiagnosis and mistreatment. Natural remedies are also outside the realm of their knowledge and therefore met with contempt and disapproval.

This 'closed mind' response from the medical profession, is not in our best interest.

The information is out there. To be fair, doctors are probably too 'flat out' busy to look for it, struggling to keep up with new drugs continually being developed or perhaps they just haven't looked hard enough. I can't answer for them. I do know that powerful pharmaceutical companies help to fund and shape their training content. This may explain their limited knowledge of nutrition and its impact on health. It would also explain the ease and readiness with which prescriptions are handed out.

On many occasions over the last 30 years I've seen individual children suffering with some illness that could have been prevented or remedied with the appropriate vitamin intake. It was distressing for the child, distressing for the mother (or ignored) and disturbing for me to see. I *knew* what the child needed to correct the situation. Sometimes I offered a solution (and I mean gently offered a solution) and gave them the name and author of my information source. Some Mothers were grateful for the help, and some drifted back into the land of Inertia.

I cannot speak for other people but as a mother, if I had to '... move heaven and earth' for my kids, I did. If I found conventional medicine didn't work (get the results) then I looked for alternatives. My children grew up and developed without any allergies. They avoided the childhood conditions that many mothers are led to believe are 'normal.' I achieved this by practicing applied nutrition from conception, to right through adolescence. Up until my 30 year old son married, I continued to put vitamins out every morning on the bench top for him to take.

TIP NUMBER TWO: YOU NEED TO BE INFORMED

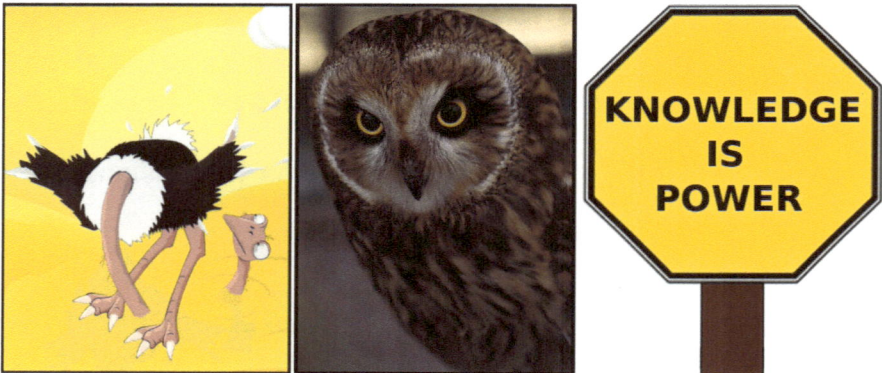

Are you like the ostrich or wise like the owl?

We don't need a degree. Not everyone has the inclination or money to go to university. The measure and value of what I've learned about nutrition over the past 30 years far out weighs the knowledge and experience found in a 4 year degree. **We DO need information** however. What we need are basic facts that are easy to find, easy to follow and to put into practice. We need to educate ourselves about vitamins/nutrients, what their role is and how they affect our health. We still need protein, carbohydrates, fats, minerals, vitamins and water etc, to function. There are also many lesser known nutrients outside of these groups.

It's the 'how much, how often and why' information that makes some of us hesitate. Why? <u>Yet we readily accept prescribed drugs that we know little or nothing about, from Physicians, without question or hesitation.</u> It is well documented that thousands (literally) of people die each year from prescription drugs. *That fact alone should have us asking questions. But we don't. Why?* For decades, we have been smoothly and skillfully conditioned. Manipulative advertising, put forth by the powerful pharmaceutical companies who produce these drugs, has taken advantage of our naivety and lack of knowledge. So, if physicians prescribe them, they must be okay…right? Not necessarily.

When I started out, I didn't have the how much, how often, information about vitamins either, but I didn't let that stop me. I checked examples and the quantities that were used in case studies and followed the advice of a renowned nutritionist. I worked from that starting point. I was simply a mother determined to help my children. I learned over time, and through experience, what dosages were effective, whether they needed to be increased, when it was okay to decrease and what combinations of nutrients were needed by monitoring responses. These things varied depending upon the severity of the illness in question and the age of the child. Nutrition is a science. Like Biology, it can be learned by anyone, and frankly, I found the effort well worth it.

Although my key source of information has long been out of print and its author no longer with us, the knowledge continues to be valuable for Mothers with growing children today. At one time, my adult son exclaimed, "Yeah but that information is years old. There's got to be more recent research and up to date information than that!" My response was, "Yes, of course there is, but human bodies still need the same nutrients today that they needed thirty, fifty or a hundred years ago. That doesn't change." Because of the changes in our environment however, the urgency and quantity of nutrients required, has increased dramatically though. And guess what; remedies that worked centuries ago, still work today. So why re invent the wheel? Conversely, it is also true that deficiencies that caused ill health long ago *still cause ill health today.* This is simple logic.

When my daughter was in year 12 in high school she was able to tell the class more fully what the role of Vitamin E entailed, because the teacher did not know. This is no discredit to the teacher, but simply to point out the need for people to do their own research and find the answers. At no time did I force feed my family with information, I taught by example. Applied nutrition became a natural family dynamic that my children grew up with.

You too can become conversant with how vitamins work, and you will be able to discern what nutrients will help your child recover from an illness, just like I have. There will come a time when you will be able to protect and prevent your child from becoming ill in the first place. I simply applied the information I had and it worked each and every time. It works for anyone who cares to use it. Including you!

It is my dearest hope that this book will help relieve the needless suffering of sick children everywhere. This book is here to lead you through the maze of uncertainty, to an understanding that will free you and empower you to take positive action and pursue good health for your family.

TIP NUMBER 3:   YOU NEED A GUIDE…

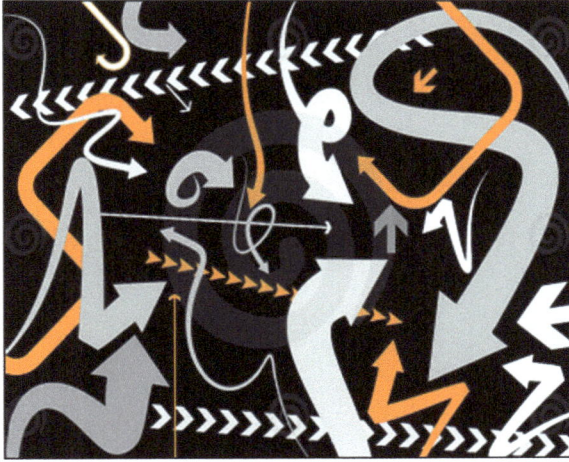

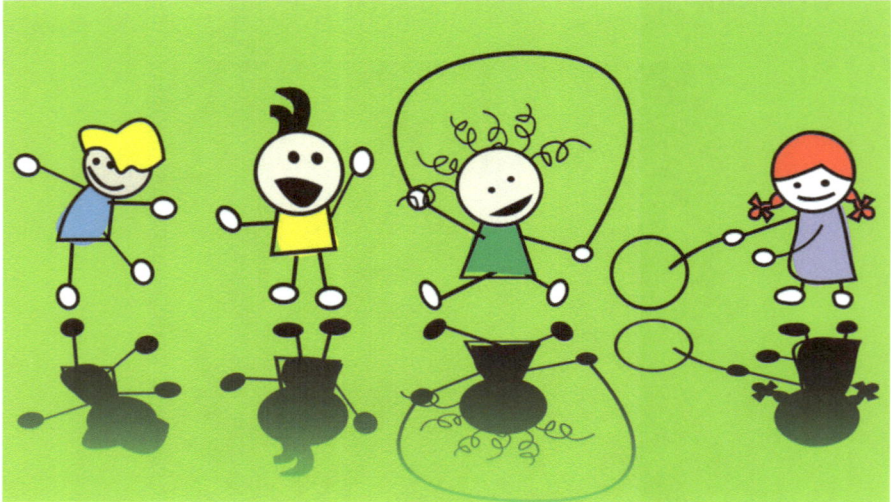

Chapter 3 – ANSWERS WHEN YOU NEED THEM A – A

ADRENAL EXHAUSTION   A

What's that you say? . . . Read on.

Adrenal exhaustion is when the adrenal glands are exhausted. It is a common condition, (very often covert), that leaves your children vulnerable to all kinds of illness and disease, especially during their early years of development and when the adrenal glands play an important role in the functioning of the immune system. Adults too, often suffer with adrenal exhaustion.

SYMPTOMS:

- During infancy, an example of adrenal exhaustion is when your baby is teething. At first he gets a cold because the stress of teething has weakened his resistance, and then he might get an ear or throat infection. Before long he starts coming down with something else or a previous illness returns.

- This is your child's body 'telling' you that it is in di*stress*. This is a red flag 'telling' you that the body needs more nutrients—the weapons required to fight infection and to prevent this situation in the first place. The adrenal glands have more than they can handle, and need extra nutrients to fight the onset of disease and the disease itself.
- In older children, swollen adenoids, tonsils or lymph glands may become evident and are advanced symptoms of adrenal exhaustion. The following statements reveal what causes this condition.
- In a healthy individual, one of the first reactions to infection (stress) is that the lymph glands shrink in size while the adrenal hormones change protein content into sugar and fat to supply energy to the   body.
- When illness occurs, there are times when the body will go into what I call 'survival mode.' It will prioritize, borrow or manufacture nutrients from one part of the body to maintain the parts that are vital for survival.
- *The point is that it should not have to do so.*
- It is *only when the adrenal glands are exhausted* that any lymph tissue can become enlarged. A child with swollen adenoids / tonsils is suffering adrenal exhaustion. Indications: low blood sugar, a craving for sweets and has infections or allergies typical of adrenal exhaustion. This does not happen overnight. **The body reaches this state because the nutrients it needs have been inadequate or missing for too long.**
- It is worth noting at this point that sugar loaded sweets/candy, (known as 'lollies' in Australia) can actually undermine and weaken the immune system. I recommend cutting back on these.
- Even when antibiotics are prescribed by the doctor, continue giving supplements—especially vitamin C
- (500mg of vitamin C with every dose of antibiotics). Antibiotics treat the symptoms, which are a good thing, but

they don't treat the cause. And if we don't treat the cause at the same time, there is nothing to prevent a relapse or stop the infection from returning.

During times of sickness the body's need for nutrients is multiplied.

REMEDY:

- Vitamin C and Pantothenic Acid (Vitamin B5) are always needed during any illness, but do not rely on these two alone. Although these two nutrients are key anti-stress vitamins, sickness of any kind is a red alert for more of *every* nutrient. Before surgery is considered, for example, an anti-stress supplement program is suggested for two or more months prior to the event, to prepare your child physically and emotionally for surgery and to hasten recovery.
- Any illness to the body is a form of stress.
- Pregnancy itself is a form of stress and this supplement program is covered in chapter 6.
- An effective program is one that supplies necessary vitamins that the body urgently needs.

My children were given the following during times of illness or stress:

Supplement Guide No 1: Explained

- 25 mg to 30 mg of **Pantothenic Acid** (Vitamin B5) 3 times a day for 2 – 3 weeks, then 2 times a day afterwards. The dosage was gradually reduced after all symptoms disappeared, to twice a day then once a day. A maintenance dose 25 mg–50 mg per day throughout childhood was given as a protective measure with 500 mg of Vitamin C.
- At any sign of illness, the dosage of 25–50mgs of Vitamin B5 (Pantothenic Acid) was increased in frequency and given *3* times per day. At the same time, *250–500*

mgs *of* Vitamin C was given, 3–4 times per day (depending on the severity of an illness), for 1–2 weeks, then reduced to 2 times per day afterwards. (A 500 mg dose taken daily is merely a maintenance dosage and a protective measure throughout childhood.)

- One Vitamin B complex tablet (chewable/crushable/dissolvable) for children each day. In my experience any supplement containing less than 10 mg to 15 mg of the key B Vitamins is simply not enough to be effective. It is a waste of money.
- I used an effervescent vitamin tablet that dissolves in water and is fruit flavored, as a supplement for my children from infancy. They drank it throughout any given day in addition to breast-feeding.
- One Cod Liver Oil capsule was given daily [for Vitamins A & D] during illness and continued after recovery. When I ceased breast feeding, 1–2 Cod Liver Oil capsules per day were given. If you miss a day, don't worry. Vitamins A & D are stored in the body; so just continue them the next day.
- One 500 IU natural Vitamin E capsule was given 3–4 times per week for sickness and maintenance.
- Because Vitamin E is generally not found in the Western diet due to processed foods; it is the most neglected vitamin.
- The above practice has proven most effective in keeping my family healthy.

Supplement Guide No: 2 Explained

Recently, I discovered a supplement called 'Nature's Way' 'Stress and fatigue fighter B' that acts as an excellent multivitamin for children and adults.

For parents outside of Australia, I have included a table of contents, so that you can match them as closely as possible with what is available in your location.

- These tablets are more easily accepted by children when mixed with a little fruit juice, fruit puree, or jam.

- They contain an ideal amount of nutrients that can be managed & measured easily.
- They are reasonably priced and good value for your money.
- They actually contain enough potency to be effective. There are so many children's supplements available that don't deliver the results.
- I shake my head in disgust at some of the supplements manufactured for children. When I see only 2 mg or 3 mg of *any* vitamin on the label, I think: 'That's okay—for a flea.'

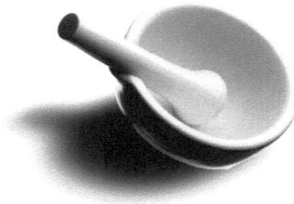

This multi-vitamin needs to be ground finely (using a mortar and pestle above) with orange/lemon flavored Vitamin C. This may be added to a desert spoon of fruit juice or puree and given by using a syringe and squirting portions of the contents into your infant or child's mouth with day-time feeds.

- This guide has been successfully used for sick infants.
- Once the condition improves and symptoms have gone, ½ a tablet per day may be enough for a daily maintenance dose. If symptoms linger, increase Vitamin B5 (Pantothenic Acid) and Vitamin C, in addition to one 'Nature's Way Stress and fatigue fighter tablet.'
- The words 'may be enough' are used simply because every individual's needs, genes, body chemistry plus the severity of the illness varies. This causes the 'how much' factor to vary as well.
- You will need to tune in to how your child responds to the nutrients. Ninety-five percent of the time I found improvement within 8 to 12 hrs irrespective of which option

is used. Sometimes recovery was quicker. Sometimes it was longer.

- If symptoms appeared not to be getting any worse but a little too slow to disappear, I would increase Vitamin C and Vitamin B5, until they disappeared, and continued this for 3–4 days after. A maintenance dose of all vitamins needs to be continued.

Contents of both supplement guides:

'Berocca B': Supplies B complex plus C

- ➢ Vitamin B1 . . . . 15 mg
- ➢ Vitamin B2 . . . . 15 mg
- ➢ Nicotinamide/Niacin (B3) . . . . .50 mg
- ➢ Pantothenic Acid (B5) . . . . 23 mg
- ➢ Vitamin B6 . . . . 10 mg
- ➢ Vitamin B12 . . . . 10 mcg
- ➢ Vitamin C . . . . 500 mg
- ➢ Biotin . . . . 150 mcg
- ➢ Folic Acid . . . . 400 mcg
- ➢ Calcium . . . . 100 mg
- ➢ Magnesium . . . . 100 mg
- ➢ Zinc . . . . 10 mg
- ➢ An extra 5 mg of Vitamin B6 needs to be added to balance Vitamin B2 and Vitamin B6 quantities.

[Note: I always check to ensure these two vitamins (B2 & B6) are the same quantity as prolonged use of an unbalanced amount in these two vitamins can cause a deficiency in the one with the lesser amount.]

'Nature's Way Stress & Fatigue Fighter' : Supplies A, B, C, D, & E plus Calcium, Zinc & Magnesium.

- ➢ Vitamin B1 . . . . 20 mg
- ➢ Vitamin B2 . . . . 25 mg
- ➢ Nicotinamide/Niacin (B3) . . . . 100 mg
- ➢ Pantothenic Acid (B5) . . . . 68.7 mg
- ➢ Pyridoxine B6 . . . . 25 mg
- ➢ Folic Acid . . . . 250 mcg
- ➢ Cyancobalamin B12 . . . . 50 mcg
- ➢ Biotin . . . . 100 mcg
- ➢ Choline . . . . 50 mg
- ➢ Inositol . . . . 50 mg
- ➢ Abscorbic Acid (Vitamin C) . . . . 150 mg
- ➢ Magnesium . . . . 30 mg
- ➢ Retinal Acetate (Vitamin A) . . . . 1000 IU
- ➢ Cholecalciferol (Vitamin D3) . . . . 2.5 mcg
- ➢ D alpha tocopherol acetate (Vitamin E) . . . . . . 30 mg

Note: mcg = micrograms

- If you use this supplement or one similar, then you will need to monitor it when consuming them in conjunction with others. As explained ahead.
- Normally, 1–2 Cod Liver Oil capsules daily [for Vitamins A & D] throughout infancy and childhood are enough for every day maintenance. If using, a supplement like "Nature's Way Stress & Fatigue Fighter" supplement which already contains Vitamin A & D in *water soluble form,* an addition of 1 Cod liver oil capsule daily may suffice. Case studies have proven that 2 tablespoons of cod liver oil can be taken daily with no toxic effects. I gave my chil-

dren 1 capsule daily or two if illness threatened and right through childhood, using a simple method of piercing the capsule and squeezing it into their mouths.

- Since Cod Liver Oil offers Vitamin A & D in its *natural form*, and is more effective than the water soluble kind, it can be given with the "Nature's Way" style supplement.

- The Nature's Way tablet can be halved, crushed and added to juice. However, during the entire teething stage and when illness threatens, ½ in the morning and ½ at night is needed to strengthen the immune system. I would also continue with Vitamin C and B5 in between on the 'teeth cutting' days. It is a good idea to keep a separate supply of Pantothenic Acid (Vitamin B5) on its own and use it as required with Vitamin C, as a top up during times of stress and/or illness.

- All the fat soluble Vitamins (A, D & E) are more effective in their natural form as opposed to the water soluble kind in the previous supplement. 500 IU's of Natural Vitamin E then, in the form of oil in capsules, can be given 3 or 4 times per week in addition to the 'Natures Way' supplement.

- Vitamins A, D and E are fat soluble vitamins which are stored in the body. Water soluble vitamins (B complex and C) are not stored—what the body does not use is passed out in urine.

- Keep in mind that while your child is on a 'maintenance dose' (after recovery), he or she is only getting half the contents of the "Nature's Way" supplement per day. But whenever illness threatens full dosage is recommended for the body's increased needs.

- The above practice has proven effective for me and my family. [We do get Vitamin A from the sun light, but each time we bathe or shower, some of it is washed off along with our natural body oils because it is a fat soluble vitamin.]

- One 500 IU Vitamin E capsule alternate days during sickness is recommended. Then continue this even when symptoms disappear. Since Vitamin E is not found in our processed western diet, this action needs to be maintained throughout childhood and upwards.

- Because Vitamins B and C are water soluble, this means that the body can tolerate high dosages or frequent smaller ones.
- These supplements may be continued for a week *after* the symptoms have stopped and then changed to a **maintenance dose.**
- It has been my practice to continue giving the above supplements especially when antibiotics are prescribed by the doctor. ** An Antibiotic will treat the symptoms, which is a good thing, but it doesn't treat the cause. And as previously mentioned, there is nothing to stop the infection/illness from returning, if you don't treat the cause at the same time. **Extra Vitamin C (500mg) needs to be taken with any medication.
- Continue supplements *after* the antibiotics are finished. Just because the symptoms have gone does not mean we stop the supplements—the body needs nutrients **ALL** the time, especially during the recovery process.

A Maintenance Dose: for Supplement Guide No: 1

One 500 mg Vitamin C and 25 mg Pantothenic Acid (Vitamin B5) **per day**, as well as 1 Cod Liver Oil capsule daily and 1 Vitamin E capsule 500 IU, 2 or 3 times per week, for children of any age.

If you are bottle feeding a B complex supplement will be needed morning and evening. Breast feeding mothers who take B complex supplements will supply these in their milk, but a boost of ½ a Berocca B tablet, fruit flavored and dissolved in water, once per day, is beneficial.

- A full range of **all** nutrients is advisable as a supplement for women during pregnancy and breast feeding.

In today's society we need a full range of supplements throughout our entire life, to maintain good health.

A Maintenance Dose : for Supplement Guide No: 2

- One "Nature's Way Stress & Fatigue Fighter," plus 500 mg Vitamin C crushed and added to water or juice, given in small portion doses with feeds—enough to cover a 2 day period.

This means the supplements are processed every 2 days so that ½ the quantity is given during day 1 and the other half during day 2.

- **During sickness a full dose is given every day until symptoms disappear completely,** and is then reverted back to a maintenance dose again.

My grandson, at 6 months old and my grand daughter 2 yrs older have responded well to the second supplement guide, and continue to do so with effective results.

Cheryl Gi

If you cannot afford all the above supplements all the time, then Vitamin C, Pantothenic Acid (Vitamin B5) when given every day, will provide *some* support to the immune system in fighting any infection/illness. These nutrients will not compensate for all the others, but they will help tide the body over for a short time, until you can afford the full quota of vitamins. If possible, include Cod Liver Oil capsules for Vitamins A & D.

The body is truly amazing. When it is constantly given all the nutrients it needs to function efficiently, illness and disease are avoided. Our body has the ability to protect itself, heal itself, maintain itself, prioritize and improvise to keep us alive and functioning. Whether our level of functioning is high or low, is entirely dependent upon the nutrients we give it. Drugs will never replace the value of nutrients.

ALLERGIES

Over 20% of our children suffer with allergies and that number is increasing rapidly. These allergies result from foreign substances, usually microscopic protein particles that gain access to the blood. Allergies can be triggered by introducing solids too early to your child's immature digestive system. Fluoridated water has also been identified as a cause of allergies.

The foreign particles mentioned enter in the following ways:
- Drug injections, vaccines and serums through the skin
- With cosmetics, insect venoms, poison ivy
- Through the mucous membranes in nasal passages
- With pollens, dust, dandruff
- The intestinal tract
- From foods, bacteria, moulds, histamine & medications

SYMPTOMS / EXPLANATION

The reaction to these substances may appear in the form of a skin rash, eczema, hives, hay fever, asthma, headaches runny/stuffy noses teary eyes, sneezing, sinus 'infections' fever and digestive disturbances or life threatening affects.

Instead of avoiding offending substances, the emphasis should be placed on building a healthy immune system. A truly healthy individual is not affected when exposed to 'allergens.'

Allergies are one of the conditions that result from having adrenal exhaustion (mentioned previously), and they are the body's reaction to stress. Stress can be the result of inadequate diet, emotional upsets, not enough sleep, infections, or the use of drugs/medications and are usually preceded by the onset of allergies. Make sure plenty of water is given daily.

Do not overlook the impact of emotional stress. Children harboring negative emotions need to find a way of releasing them, or it will find release through their body. The added stress of a toxic allergen is the 'straw that breaks the camel's back.'

Stress on its own increases the body's need for almost every nutrient.

People suffering from allergies have been found to be woefully deficient in every nutrient, except carbohydrates and when these missing nutrients have been supplied the allergies have often disappeared.

The adrenal cortex is extremely sensitive to being deprived of nutrients. A deficiency of B5 (Pantothenic Acid) alone, causes the glands to shrivel and to become filled with blood and dead cells, so that cortisone and other hormones can no longer be produced or function. This leaves the body vulnerable. There is not a single part of your body that is not affected by hormones. Not enough Linoleic Acid, Vitamin A, B2, E, or Essential Fatty Acids, has the same effect of vulnerability or risk.

I hope you are beginning to see the importance of supplementing your diet with a potent _ALL inclusive_ set of nutrients. Each one of them works in conjunction with others. For example, when taking Calcium the body will not absorb it unless sufficient Magnesium and Vitamin D is taken with it. Vitamin C also contributes to Calcium functioning. Without these supportive nutrients, Calcium is passed out in urine and is wasted.

I could write a whole chapter on how nutrients interact with each other and how to maximize their effectiveness from that perspective but I want to avoid 'information overload'.

(Should you wish to understand in more depth, how nutrients interact with each other my contact details are supplied on the final page.) Instead, I will expand on them a little as I come to discuss each one in this format.

Case Studies:

Children suffering from asthma, hives, or eczema have improved dramatically when the only change to their diet was the addition of Cod liver oil and a supplement of B12. According to Davis, a study of 32 children with allergies was made, in an attempt to give them an 'adequate' diet. This group, who suffered from bronchial asthma and allergic eczema, were given generous amounts of protein, NO refined carbohydrates, and adequate essential fatty acids.

A daily supplement of 600 mg of Vitamin C, 32 mg (Note that 'mg' = milligrams and differs from IU = international units) of vitamin E, 20,000 IU of Vitamin A, 800 IU of Vitamin D and moderate amounts of B complex vitamins, was also included. **Within one single month most of these young children had recovered, and within two months all of them had.**

Allergies have been produced repeatedly in animals by injections of foreign substances. The reaction appeared to be more severe and in some cases, fatal when B5 (Pantothenic Acid) was deficient.

When people who normally suffered with severe hay fever were given cortisone before being exposed to pollens, they did not suffer the disease. Wait! There is no need to go to the doctor to get a cortisone injection!

THE BODY PRODUCES ITS *OWN* CORTISONE WHEN WE GIVE IT THE NUTRIENTS IT NEEDS TO FUNCTION CORRECTLY!

During an asthma attack, a group of patients (adults) were given 300 mg of Vitamin C every 15 minutes. Some experienced immediate relief and others within the hour. Further attacks were prevented when 15,000 mg of Vitamin C were taken daily.

In a study where 50 babies with skin rashes were labeled as being allergic to milk, none showed improvement when milk intake was stopped. These rashes are usually caused by a lack of B Vitamins or Linoleic Acid, and have cleared up when the missing nutrients were supplied.

Healthy cells can prevent allergens from entering the body. A lack of almost any nutrient can weaken cell structure and allow allergens in. Not only that, but bacteria and viruses also enter.

Vitamin A has an especially strong role in protecting the cell walls to prevent allergens, bacteria, viruses or toxic substances from entering the body. However, it does its best work when Vitamin E and all other nutrients are present in sufficient quantities.

Giving babies solid foods before the digestive tract is mature enough to handle them, can contribute to food allergies, in children. The most common allergy is to wheat. With any indication of a food allergy e.g. to milk or wheat, introduce enzymes with every meal to assist digestion and recovery.

When an inherited (hereditary) allergy appears, special efforts should be made to breast feed an infant. It follows that you the mother need to take supplements to compensate for the inherited deficiencies that contribute to this condition and give supplements to your baby as well as yourself.

[Case studies taken from *Let's Get Well*, by Adelle Davis, pages 193-204]

REMEDY:

The supplement regime found under Adrenal Exhaustion in Chapter 1, with extra Vitamin C depending upon the severity of the illness, will reduce symptoms.

The Supplement Guide No: 2 compares well with the Asthma case studies previously mentioned.

"Supplements in today's world are an absolute re-

quirement, as we no longer receive an adequate supply from our food. Be aware that nutrients do not act alone nor do they have only one type of action in the body. This is why it is vitally important that we need to take a full range of nutritional supplementation".

Dr. Alex Omelchuk

ANEMIA

SYMPTOMS/ EXPLANATION:

Anemia has many causes. It is the result of the oxygen carrying hemoglobin in the blood cells being in short supply. Healthy blood cells are produced in the bone marrow provided that ample raw materials (nutrients) are supplied. Anemia exists when the red cell count is less than 80%. Since little oxygen reaches the tissues during this condition, energy cannot be produced. Constant tiredness, lack of stamina, pallor, shortness of breath and sometimes dizziness, headaches and depression can result.

Iron deficiency is the most well-known cause of anemia. However, it can also be caused by the following:
- Vitamin B6 deficiency anemia
- Vitamin E deficiency anemia
- Folic Acid deficiency anemia.
- A lack of stomach acid can induce anemia (when the key B complex vitamins are deficient.)
- Affect of drugs and insecticides can destroy Vitamin E and induce anemia.

REMEDY:

Do not assume that an iron deficiency may be the cause and take iron supplements without professional advice.

Have your naturopath/health professional conduct blood tests to check the above factors. An excess of Iron may be rare, but can cause other complications.

Taking a well-balanced range of all nutrients as demonstrated in Supplement Guide No: 2, (under Adrenal Exhaustion), is a safe way to go, this supports the body's recuperative powers and promotes good health maintenance.

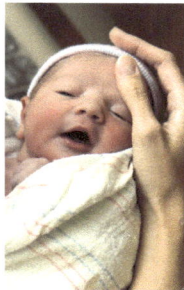

ARTHRITIS

SYMPTOMS / EXPLANATION:

Arthritis is another disease that is rapidly increasing in people of all ages. It produces a crippling pain in the joints, making it difficult to sleep and affects the ability to function.

There have been cases where an infant as young as 6 months, a 4 and a 5 year old, as well as a 15 year old, having arthritis. All of these children responded to an adequate diet and nutrient intake. Obviously their diet had been *in*adequate before.

This illness can be avoided by making sure your child's intake of nutrients is high enough and maintained on a daily basis. In the case of the infant, breast feeding with a nutritionally vigilant mother who took daily supplements, plus a maintenance supplement for the infant would have been beneficial.

REMEDY:

Drink lots of pure water, specifically water, avoid high acid foods and take high potency vitamin supplements. See an example below. Do not expect an overnight response—this will take time. Apart from a number of herbal supplements obtained from Health shops that ease arthritis, there are other remedies. Below are a few that have achieved remarkable results.

- Avoid white carbohydrates e.g. white rice, flour, bread, pasta, sugar etc and foods highly acidic.
- Pycnogenol Is a supplement extracted from the bark of a French Maritime Pine tree species, combined with several bioflavonoids and fruit acids.
- Its numerous studies and results are well documented and it has many healing properties. Pycnogenol is a powerful antioxidant and anti inflammatory which can relieve joint pain /arthritis.
- Cherries: eat 6 per day or 4 ounces of cherry juice. I have viewed over 35 testimonies from people who have achieved excellent results using cherries/juice.
- Turmeric has strong anti inflammatory action.
- Apple cider vinegar in water has been successful for many. About I tablespoon of cider vinegar mixed (with ½ teaspoon of honey if desired) in a glass of water and taken with every meal. This keeps calcium in solution form and prevents it from lodging in the body's tissues.
- By combining a number of approaches at the same time, e.g. modifying diet, taking antioxidants, natural anti inflammatory supplements and lots of water, the results will be more effective. Recovery takes time.

Personal Case Study:

When my son was diagnosed with arthritis at 10 years old, I was deeply concerned and shocked. Perhaps the fast foods and cola syndrome sneaked up on me, or maybe it was caused through an inherited deficiency. Anyway it was a wake up call for me to be more vigilant. He was my third child and maybe I had become a little complacent.

I modified his diet to avoid foods high in acid and increased his vitamins and water intake, especially Vitamin C which is a natural anti-inflammatory plus anti-histamine, antibiotic, anti-toxin. Vitamin E also acts as an anti inflammatory and was also given.

He took prescribed anti-inflammatory medication coupled with 500mg of Vitamin C with each prescription dose. After a few months he was able to reduce the medication and the arthritic attacks became milder, fewer and far between. Within 10–12 months he was able to stop the medication altogether, but I continued to monitor his diet and supplements.

Since that time he has not had a recurrence, he eats without having to avoid certain foods, and he keeps a check on his eating habits.

Cheryl G.

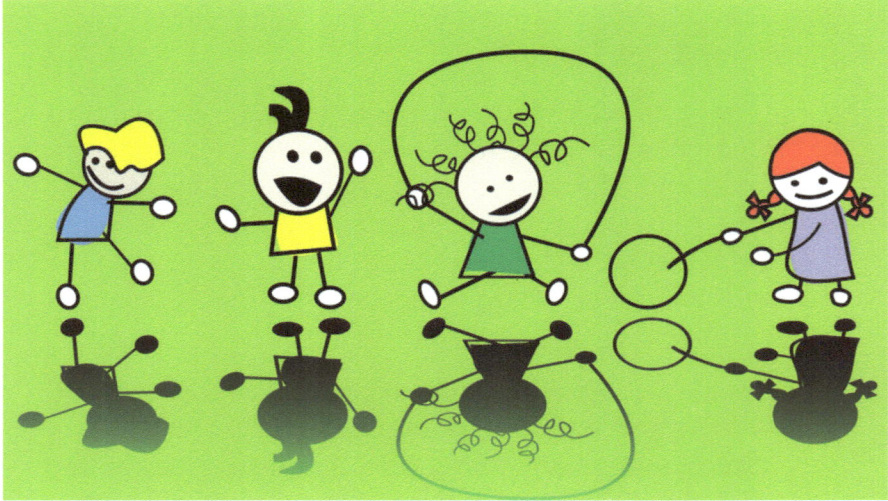

Chapter 4 – ANSWERS WHEN YOU NEED THEM B – C

BILIRUBIN: commonly known as JAUNDICE B

SYMPTOMS:

- Jaundice explained: Bilirubin is a natural and continuous body process for worn-out red blood cells that need to be disposed of.
- During this process the coloring matter of these cells forms a pigment called bilirubin, which is usually excreted in bile soon after it is formed. When Vitamin E is deficient however, many blood cells are destroyed so rapidly that this pigment cannot be expelled quickly enough.
- It then accumulates and settles into the tissues causing the baby to become jaundiced. I.e. the baby's skin has a sickly, yellow tinge. The healthy pink pictured is desirable.

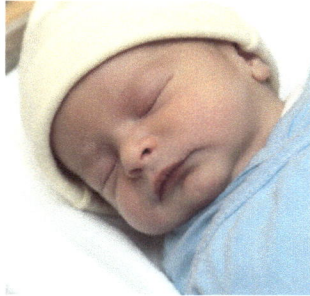

REMEDY:

The remedy of course is to supply Vitamin E. The most effective results are achieved by:

- Squeezing the contents of a 500 IU Vitamin E capsule directly into the baby's mouth once per day at feeding time, for 2–3 days. If the capsule quantity appears to be too much to swallow in one dose, then squeeze ½ the contents in one feed and the other ½ in the next feed.
- At the same time you, the mother, need to increase your Vitamin E intake to 1000 IU per day for one week and continue taking at least 500 IU during the breast feeding period. When breast feeding stopped, 500 IU daily as a maintenance dose has been my practice.
- Assuming you are breastfeeding, frequent feeds during the first 3 days also assist in correcting the problem. After the first week, a maintenance dose of 500 IU daily [or 1,000 IU alternate days] by you is needed for as long as you are breast feeding.
- Avoid baby formula that contains Iron; try using goat's milk or full cream cow's milk (organic) with the Vitamin E. **The Iron in formula destroys Vitamin E and defeats the purpose.**
- Vitamin E needs to be taken 9–10 hours after Iron because Iron prevents Vitamin E from doing its job if taken at the same time. Avoid iron and Vitamin E meeting each other in the digestive system.

BITES, STINGS AND SCRATCHES

SYMPTOMS:

- Bee stings, insect bites and scratches can become inflamed, itchy and swollen. Some have a toxic or allergic reaction for some people. These minor wounds can also become infected. In the case of a toxic or allergic reaction there may be difficulty in breathing. More children die from allergies to bee stings than being bitten from poisonous snakes.
- Using a bee sting as an example: Whether you escape to the country or stay tucked away in a well-manicured backyard, you are bound to have a close encounter with a bee a few times in your life.
- Bee stings can be painful at best, and fatal if you're allergic to them. Fortunately, only four percent of the human population is allergic to bee stings, which means you probably won't require medical attention. Even if you're not allergic, you can reduce the pain and swelling if you respond correctly to this little trauma, with a swift removal of the stinger. Current research indicates a swift removal is best.
- After a bee stings you and deposits its stinger, the stinger continues to pump venom into your bloodstream for up to 20 minutes. A self-contained unit, the stinger has a barb to pierce your skin, a venom sac to hold the stuff that stings you, and a set of muscles to push the barb and venom deeper into your skin.

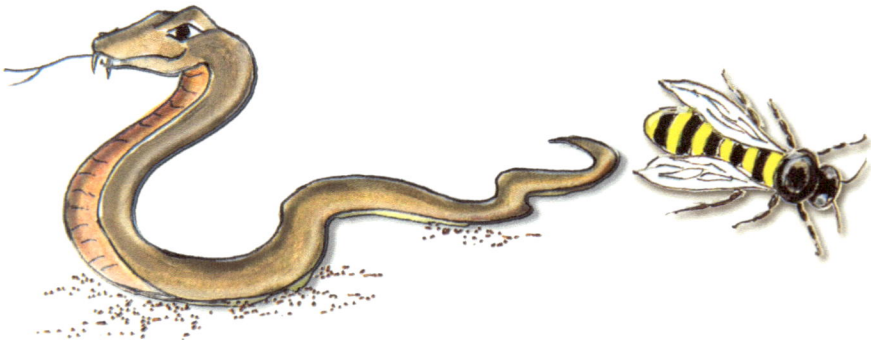

REMEDY:

Scorpion stings, wasp stings, black widow spider bites, rattle snake bites and others have been treated successfully by Dr. Fred Klenner, with an injection of 1,000 mg of Vitamin C.

- Vitamin C is a natural anti-toxin and can be given orally for a bite or sting of this nature. It is absorbed into the body quite quickly.
- It is important to initially build up to a 500–1000 mg dose of Vitamin C before hand and then keep to this amount (500mg) as a daily maintenance dose. Why?
- Because you cannot anticipate when your child may re-act to a bite or sting of this nature, and a sudden dose of 1,000 mg orally, may not be processed effectively when the body is not used to it and can cause a loose bowel movement.
- The 500 mg per day action also protects and prepares the body for any contingency—any infection or crisis that requires mega-doses.
- The second benefit is that the Vitamin C coupled with an already strong immune system (which you have main-tained), helps to **prevent** a reaction so that it does not develop into an allergy.
- **If your child develops breathing difficulties, any swelling around eyes, lips, tongue or genitals, any red blotching, light-headedness or fainting, then they must be seen by a doctor immediately**.
- My children were all given 500 mg or more of Vitamin C daily as a safety measure.
- Mosquito bites often leave an itchy lump that is eased by the anti-histamine action of Vitamin C, when taken orally and sprayed onto the wound (see page 52).
- Tea Tree antiseptic cream can be applied to the skin.
- I automatically follow my own advice with 1,000 mg or more daily of Vitamin C.
- A little vinegar or a mixture of baking soda and water may be applied to ease the soreness of the area.

BLOCKED TEAR DUCT (or 'sticky eye')

SYMPTOMS:

- About half of all babies develop a blocked tear duct some time in the first 3 months after birth. Because it is not a severe problem, parents are usually not given a clear explanation. Most sticky eyes in young babies are caused by a blockage in the ducts which drain the eye.
- This is generally caused through the soft tissues being cramped.
- The facial bones have not formed to their full capacity due to poor Calcium absorption and have not allowed the space required for the tear ducts to function properly. Hence they become blocked.

REMEDY:

- If a breastfeeding mother increases her Calcium combined with magnesium and Vitamin D, it will be released into her milk.
- One Cod Liver Oil capsule per day, for one week and then continued alternate days – for an infant, will ensure good Calcium absorption and promote fully developed bone structure in a breast-fed baby.
- In a bottle-fed baby it is necessary to rely heavily on supplements, e.g. the Supplement Guide No: 2.
- In the mean time, gently clean the eyes with a saline solution which can be purchased from any pharmacy.

NOTE: This is not to be confused with conjunctivitis (pictured). Conjunctivitis makes eyes feel gritty, sore and expels pus from the inflamed eyes. This needs to be seen by a doctor. It is contagious and can be bacterial or viral.

Blocked tear ducts do not have these symptoms.

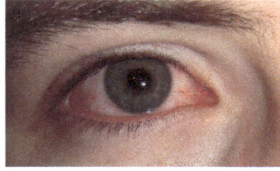
Conjunctivitis

BURNS

SYMPTOMS:

- The agonizing pain associated with burns appears to result from a lack of oxygen in that area, as the supply of this is cut off the moment blood vessels are seared. The pain continues as the heat from the burn continues to 'cook.' Blisters may occur and the wound becomes sensitive to the touch.

REMEDY:

- Apply cold running water for minor burns or a cold pack (a packet of frozen peas will do) to take the heat out of the wound. First Aid instructs us to seek medical advice for any burn the size of a 20 cent piece or bigger.
- Because the damaged tissues release toxic-breakdown-products into the blood, large amounts of Vitamin C, B5 and other B complex vitamins are needed plus Calcium Gluconate on an hourly basis for 2 or 3 days with a severe burn. Pain is greatly reduced and recovery is more rapid. For a minor burn these nutrients can be given 4 times daily.
- The fluids oozing from the surface of large burns cause a huge loss of nutrients and have been known to cause death or advanced malnutrition. The extreme *stress* of a severe burn increases ALL body requirements for nutrients.
- When Vitamin E capsules are pierced with a needle and

the contents squeezed over the burned area, the pain is dulled and often disappears. More Vitamin E should be applied several times daily. About 200 IU of Vitamin E (1/3 of a 500 IU capsule) needs to be taken orally 2 or 3 times per day and 50 mg of PABA (Para Amino Benzoic Acid) while the wound is still painful. When the pain has ceased, the PABA can be discontinued but the Vitamin E needs to be daily for long after healing is complete.

- Once healing is complete 500 IU of Vitamin E can be given 2 or 3 times per week. Increase the maintenance dose of all vitamins collectively as with the onset of any illness. After 2 weeks of this, revert to maintenance dose again.

Personal Case Study: When my youngest son was about two or three years old, a hot iron fell on the back of his hand. A huge blister immediately formed. I raced out and picked some Aloe Vera plant from the garden and applied the pulp straight onto the wound. It took the pain out of the wound quickly. I applied the pulp every 20 minutes for about 2 hours, then changed to Vitamin E externally as well as orally, and continued the dosage of maintenance supplements. It healed quickly, and without infection, scarring, or a doctor's visit. I have since found an alternative treatment just as effective mentioned in the next tip.

Cheryl Gi

A Tip for Burns: Keep Vitamin C powder (or crushed tablets) in a cheap spray bottle and store it in the refrigerator. When an emergency arises quickly add sterile water to the Vitamin C powder, shake and spray directly onto the burn. Inflammation will disappear within minutes. Vitamin E applied later, will ease the pain, hasten healing and prevent scarring.

BRONCHITIS / LARENGITIS / TONSILITIS

SYMPTOMS:

A sore, raw and inflamed throat is evidence of bronchitis. Coughing can occur and thick yellow phlegm often results. Coughing hurts and comes from the bronchi at the base of the throat. The Larynx and Tonsils often join the party.

Pharyngitis, which is an infection of the pharynx or voice box, causes a person to lose their voice for a time.

REMEDY:

Bronchitis (and it's counterparts above) is a respiratory tract infection (RTI). It is a manifestation of Adrenal Exhaustion, and is discussed under that heading. Whether the infection is triggered by bacteria or viral, the body is clearly telling you it needs nutrients, lots of nutrients, **all** the nutrients, in order to fight the infection and recover.

Huge amounts of Vitamin C with B5, plus Cod Liver Oil capsules [Vitamins A & D] and B complex and Vitamin E.

[See Supplement Guide No: 2, under Adrenal Exhaustion]

As an added precaution, I have found that these infections/viruses seem to be more prevalent in the winter months. This led me to theorize that cold weather was a factor in the development of the infection. By getting your child to inhale steam it changes that environment and hastens recovery. The germs and viruses don't like the heat. The steam also helps to loosen phlegm and reduce congestion.

COLIC C

SYMPTOMS:

- Firstly, I need to clarify genuine colic from other colic-like symptoms:
- At one time or another we have all suffered some discomfort or a twinge of pain, as gas rolls around our intestines. This is not colic.
- Colic is not caused through a baby's inability to burp. This might contribute to some discomfort like the 'twinge' above, but it is short-lived.
- Genuine colic starts out like indigestion and gets more uncomfortable as time passes. It increases into an unbearable pain which can bring an adult to their knees.
- So for a baby it can be excruciating pain.
- There appears to be various causes and forms of colic that can range from mild discomfort to very painful. The medical profession has been unable to find a cause and is therefore unable to offer an effective solution.
- *Genuine colic that has a baby curling up and screaming with pain* cannot be explained, by the medical profession and the relaxing medication that may be offered by some doctors is not the answer. It may keep the baby quiet, because the infant is drugged, but it only offers temporary relief and does not treat the cause. It is distressing for both baby and parents.
- Your baby has been fed through the umbilical cord during the 9 months of pregnancy. Not through it's mouth. It makes sense then that your baby's digestive system might need to get used to the idea of processing food.
- The digestive system needs time to mature.
- Some baby's appear to cope with this task initially and some don't. When they don't process the food well enough it causes the undigested food to produce bacteria (ferment) in the bowel and the gas that forms from this causes distension and pain. The gas released from the bowel has a foul smell because of this fermented food.

- Colic symptoms tend to peak (get worse) in the afternoon and evening because earlier feeds have left a portion of undigested food which has accumulated.
- Not enough Potassium can induce colic and digestive disturbance.
- A lack of B Vitamins interferes with digestion and can also contribute to colic.
- Pain labeled as colic can also be caused through intestinal cramps which result from a deficiency of Magnesium, Calcium or Vitamin B6.

REMEDY:

- The first thing to do is to support your baby's digestive system with an enzyme supplement. Enzymes help break down the food. Normally the body produces its own enzymes, but in this case, your baby is struggling and needs assistance. Papaya enzymes (or other pleasant tasting ones) for example, can be purchased at chemists' and health shops.
- For the first 3 days crush 7 Enzyme tablets and 2 x 50 mg Pantothenic Acid (B5) tablets.
- Mix this into about 50 mg of water, using a syringe squeeze 10 ml into the side of your baby's mouth just before, or during, each feeding. The amount prepared should be enough to cover day and night feedings for 1 day. You will notice a reduction in symptoms almost straight away, on the day you start.

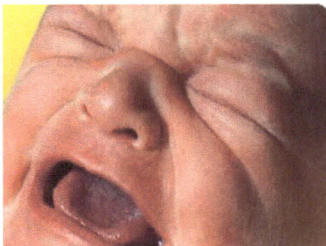

Before Enzymes/Vitamins   After Enzymes/Vitamins

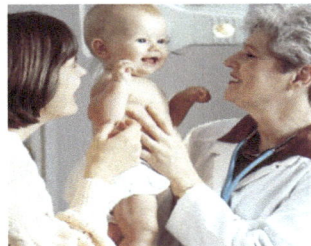

- If you are breast feeding – and it is so much easier if you are, then increase your intake of the vitamins to maximize the effectiveness.
- If bottle feeding then check to see if these nutrients are in the formula. The adding of a little extra Potassium is suggested, e.g. add ½ a 50mg Potassium tablet crushed, into the enzyme mixture above as an added precaution.
- After 2 days the dosage can be reduced to day feedings only for 2-3 days and then down to mid-day and the last feeding before bed. Monitor your baby's condition closely and give supplements as required. Usually after 4 – 5 months your baby can manage without the enzymes, **but he/she still needs vitamins.**
- Enzymes are a temporary measure to assist the body. Vitamins are needed *all* the time. Commercial baby foods tend to overlook Potassium and will remain a poor imitation of breast milk. Check contents and give supplements where necessary.
- CAUTION: Where a baby has had colic, <u>do not introduce solids earlier than 6 months</u>. A baby's digestive system is geared to handle breast milk for the first six months. *Why make their little bodies work harder than they need to and create problems?*
- *Introducing solids too early can trigger allergies.*
- An added approach that has worked for some babies with a mild form of colic is to wrap your baby firmly in a swaddling fashion using a light weight blanket / cloth. Do this after feeding and burping and before putting him down to sleep. This may work for new born babies for several weeks.
- A gentle body massage may also help sooth your baby.

Personal Case study:

Two of my three children came down with colic when they were about 2 weeks old. My first child was given papaya enzymes (tablets crushed) with each feeding. I also gave her 25 mg of Vitamin B5 (Pantothenic Acid) and 500 mg of Vitamin C mixed into the enzyme twice daily, to counter the stress.

With my third child I started out with the enzymes but then I discovered that Potassium was a possible factor, from my nutritional research.

My own health indicated a need for extra Potassium, which of course became present in my milk. Three times I ran out of Potassium and I didn't think anything of it, until my son started screaming with colic. That got my attention. I realized that the only thing different about my diet was the missing Potassium. A 25 mg tablet was crushed (mixed with a little milk/water) then given to my son in 3 doses throughout the day, for two days by spoon or syringe. This resulted in immediate relief. At the same time I resumed my intake of this mineral. *This happened three times – each time I ran out of Potassium!!

Among other things, Potassium facilitates the peristalsis process in the bowel. I made sure not to run out of it again.

All three of my children were breast-fed for 18 months and solid foods were *not* introduced until 6 months had passed. I continued to take the high dosage supplements that were my regime during pregnancy, to keep up a high quality milk supply and to maintain my own health.

Cheryl G.

CONSTIPATION

SYMPTOMS:

- Constipation is where a dry, hard stool or bowel movement is difficult and uncomfortable for your child to pass. It is not necessarily an infrequent bowel movement. It is far less likely to occur when breast feeding. Constipation can be caused by a lack of B complex vitamins, Magnesium and/or Potassium. The condition can be aggravated if not enough water or fiber is consumed.

REMEDY:

- Remove/reduce sugar from your child's diet. Have yogurt with every feed/meal and add acidophilus culture to food where ever possible. These help to create B vitamins in the bowel. A little prune juice taken may also be helpful.
- Increase leafy greens and fruit intake. Bananas are rich in potassium.
- Give your child a maintenance dose of supplements, as mentioned Supplement Guide No: 2, where B Vitamins and minerals are supplied, to avoid constipation. Giving your infant /child home made yoghurt is the best. It is pleasant to taste (not sour) and contains no sweeteners/sugar.

CRADLE CAP

SYMPTOMS:

- Infants with crusty, brownish scabs on their scalp are an indication of cradle cap. It is often mistaken for a form of dermatitis. It is caused through a deficiency in Vitamin B6. Zinc may also be a factor. Cradle cap is an indication that the infant's need for B6 is unusually high. Some need 4 to 20 times more than other children especially if the mother has been deficient in this vitamin during pregnancy. A B6 deficiency is common during pregnancy.

REMEDY:

- If your baby is being breast-fed, simply increase your B complex vitamins and take with the other essential nutrients as part of your daily routine.
- If bottle feeding, B6 and Magnesium can be added to the formula, using the supplements mentioned in Supplement Guide No: 2.
- Another option is to crush into powder, a B6 tablet and mix it with a little Zinc and *vegetable oil, and apply this frequently to the scalp. Applying it before the night-time sleep might be a more convenient time and avoids unwanted attention from others.
- To obtain the best results I would use *Cod Liver Oil or Vitamin E oil instead of the vegetable oil mentioned and continue treatment until the scalp is clear.
- When washing the scalp use a gentle soap or shampoo that does NOT contain Sodium Laurel Sulphate (or Propylene Glycol) in any form.

CROSSED-EYES

SYMPTOMS:
The following images are examples of when one or both eyes are not aligned correctly and are commonly called 'crossed' eyes. Sometimes only one eye is turned inwards.

REMEDY:

- It has been claimed that cases of cross-eyed babies have been corrected when 3,000 IU of Vitamin E were given daily.

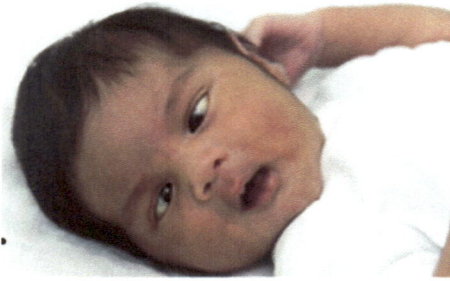

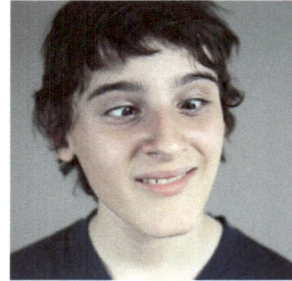

- This condition can be remedied if adequate nutrients and <u>especially Vitamin E</u> are taken during pregnancy and while breastfeeding.
- This condition is generally caused by an inherited deficiency, which could have been corrected by your ancestors but wasn't, perhaps due to lack of awareness.

Personal Case Study:

My youngest son was born with his left eye turned slightly inwards. I believed this to be a hereditary factor as there was evidence of it in my husband's family. I had been taking high potency supplements for several years.

I searched everywhere for information about this condition but could find very little. In the end I used my knowledge of vitamins and how they functioned.

I knew that Vitamin E strengthened muscle and healed soft tissue.

I gave my son 500 IU of natural Vitamin E squeezed from a capsule, daily for 2 months, then alternate days for almost a year, until the eye straightened.

It is worth noting that I also breast fed him 18 months,

which supplied extra Vitamin E. No corrective glasses or surgery was required. I was determined to avoid the eye-patch and glasses that I had seen imposed on another child with the same condition—"to strengthen the eye"!

If bottle feeding, I would give my infant one Vitamin E capsule (500 IU) 4 or 5 days per week until the eye/s straightened and avoid baby formula containing iron.

Cheryl G.

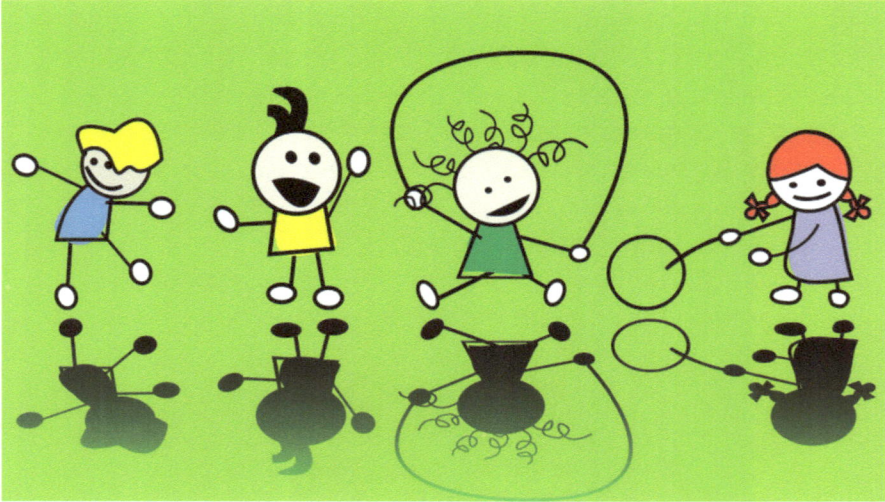

Chapter 5 – ANSWERS WHEN YOU NEED THEM D – V

DIAPER or NAPPY RASH

SYMPTOMS:

- Although nappy (diaper) rash is quite common, that doesn't mean that it's okay. Sometimes it can become quite severe and painful, raw skin develops.
- Nappy rash can be caused through disposable nappies and/or not changing nappies frequently enough. Because babies are born deficient in the fat soluble Vitamins, A, D and E, they may be more vulnerable to nappy rash. This is because fat soluble vitamins have difficulty travelling through the placenta to the infant. This can be overcome by taking water soluble Vitamin E during the final month of pregnancy. Vitamin A and E are particularly good for healthy skin and the B vitamins also contribute.

REMEDY:

- Ensure an adequate intake of Vitamin A and E is taken (by mother and baby). A recurring rash that refuses to heal may indicate an increase is required. One way to prevent nappy rash is to allow the baby to be without a nappy as often as possible.
- The important thing to remember is to remove nappies as soon as they are dirty or wet. Clean the area gently with warm water; don't put on a new nappy until skin is completely dry. Use nappies that allow the skin to breathe. Vitamin E (oil in capsules) mixed with a little Zinc cream and a few drops of Cod Liver Oil works well when applied to the affected area. A thick coating prevents urine from irritating the skin further. Calendula cream also has healing abilities and may sooth the soreness.
- **Avoid using bubble baths/soaps containing Sodium Laurel Sulphate or creams containing Propylene Glycol completely.**

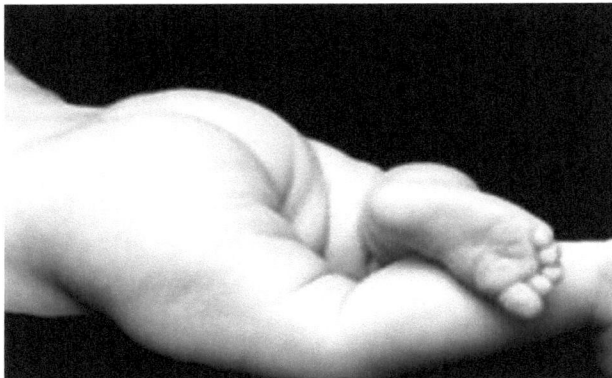

Case Study:

An Amazing Tale (No pun intended)

Recently on New Year's Eve my 2 grandchildren stayed overnight. My 2 year old grandson was in the throes of a gastric infection which caused severe inflammation and soreness on his buttocks. In spite of swift and frequent nappy changes and applying cream to the area, it became impossible to touch or clean without him screaming in pain. I ended up gently squirting his lower body with water from the garden hose to clean him, because he couldn't bear to be touched. After gently patting the area dry I pierced a double strength (1,000 IU) Vitamin E capsule and squeezed it onto the inflamed area.

This was very lightly spread over the area, left for a minute and then coated with a cream combining zinc and cod liver oil. Then a nappy was put on. The screaming prior to this treatment was reduced to a whimper and he settled for the night.

In the morning I could not believe my eyes when I went to change his nappy. I wish I had a before and after photo because I was astounded by what I saw.

I expected the Vitamin E to heal rapidly—like a day or two, but this was unbelievable! There was no inflammation, no soreness and no evidence of surface blistering.

Overnight his bottom had gone from blistering, raw skin to a smooth healthy pink with no pain or discomfort.

It was the fastest and most effective recovery I have ever seen.

Cheryl G.

ECZEMA

SYMPTOMS:

Eczema is a non-contagious skin condition that usually appears in early childhood. In some cases, eczema may continue into adulthood. The skin becomes dry, cracked and itchy, and may weep. Eczema can vary in severity and can alter daily.

REMEDY:

- Eczema occurs when babies are kept on formulas of skim milk or defatted soy milk. The lack of **Lineolic Acid** causes an infant to develop eczema or skin rashes during their first month.
- This type of eczema is corrected quickly when the baby is allowed breast milk, cow's milk, goat's milk or some vegetable oil added to their diet.
- Some short term relief can be found when vegetable oil is applied to the skin.
- **It is possible for a breast-fed baby to get eczema and indicates that the mother needs to seriously increase all supplements into her diet especially the deficiencies mentioned in the following.**
- **Any deficiency** or lack of **B complex vitamins** may cause eczema, which is common in formulas. The B Vitamins have a significant role in the absorption of fat and **Zinc,** which in turn help to rectify eczema. The absence of lactose (present in milk) also contributes to eczema.
- So it makes sense to ensure these nutrients are given to your child by breast feeding or adding separate supplements. Zinc is easily absorbed into the skin and into the blood stream by applying Zinc cream to the arm pit.
- Using goat's milk soap is also helpful. Avoid soaps with any form of Sodium Laurel Sulphate.

EPILEPSY

SYMPTOMS:

Epilepsy is characterized by recurrent, disorganized, abnormal functioning of the brain. This disruption can cause recurrent seizures. There are different kinds of seizures, and symptoms of each type can affect people differently. A seizure:
- Can last a few seconds or a few minutes
- A person can be alert or unconscious
- A person may stare into space for a few minutes or experience a few muscle twitches.
- Can cause a person to fall to the ground or make the muscles stiffen or jerk out of control – convulsions.
- Can have no warning or some people experience an aura before, to warn them.
- A 'Grand Mal' seizure has the most serious and violent convulsions.

REMEDY:

- In various case studies, physicians who have investigated epilepsy have given either magnesium OR vitamin B6. Only on rare occasions however, have they given both these nutrients together.
- One progressive physician has achieved positive results by giving epileptic children 1 teaspoon of Epsom salts in fruit juice with breakfast and 25 milligrams of vitamin B6 with every meal.
- He then discontinues all drugs after one week. He later reported that none of his young [children] patients has suffered a recurrence of epilepsy, in spite of reducing the amounts given. Note that the nutrients are continued but drugs are no longer necessary.
- If a child of mine were to suffer epilepsy I would follow these actions exactly and then continue on a maintenance level of ½ teaspoon of Epsom salts and 1 x 25mg of vitamin B6 daily.

- Please note that taking vitamin B6 separate from the other B complex vitamins on a long term basis can actually cause a deficiency in B2 if these two vitamins are not taken in balanced quantities.
- It is assumed that in the case of epilepsy it is an indication that these nutrients are in short supply to the body, and therefore need to be taken long term to avoid further attacks. To address this issue I would simply take a high potency B complex tablet and alternate this with the magnesium and B6 combination, at different times throughout each day. e.g. B complex & Magnesium at breakfast, Magnesium & B6 combination at lunch, B Complex and Magnesium at dinner and Magnesium & B6 combination at bedtime.
  [Case study taken from 'Let's Get well' by Adelle Davis, p 299]

FACIAL MALFORMATIONS: TEETH, CHIN & OTHERS.

SYMPTOMS:

- Teeth become crooked when the jaw grows incorrectly. Poor growth of the jaw will also spoil the look of the face. This can be avoided if the jaw can be encouraged to grow correctly from a young age.
- Most orthodontists are currently taught that it is too difficult to alter the growth of the jaw, or not worth the effort, and prefer the more reliable option of fixed braces, often accompanied with extractions and sometimes jaw surgery.
- If your child's face does not look quite like the other childrens', you should be concerned. Watch for flattening of the cheeks or an unusual shape around the mouth because these will almost certainly get worse. Look for dark circles under the eyes and slumping shoulders.
- **Where should the teeth be?** To measure the correct position of the upper front teeth simply put a pencil mark on the most forward point of the nose, and measure from there to the edge of the upper front teeth. Ideally it should

be 28 mm at the age of five and increase one mm each year until puberty, then it should be 38 mm to 42 mm for a girl of 16 and 40 mm to 44 mm for a boy of 17. If it is more than five millimeters over this position, there will be some irregularity of the teeth and disfigurement of the face, and if more than eight millimeters the child is certain to grow up with an unappealing face.

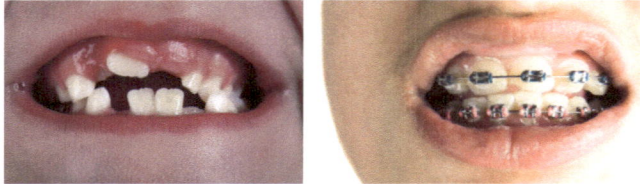

- We need to watch closely for these anomalies so that we can correct the development in time.
- **Spaces.** At the age of five there should be spaces between all front teeth. Their permanent successors which should arrive about the age of six are a lot larger, and if there is not enough space they will crowd. It is easier to prevent crowding by creating space than to correct it afterwards.
- Things like a weak or prominent chin, excessive gums, speech problems, can all be indications of poor bone development and not enough Vitamin D.
- Many attractive children grow up to lose that attractiveness when they reach adolescence and so many teenagers have to wear braces to straighten their teeth. It is sad that this expensive dental care could be avoided with 1or 2 cod liver oil capsules per day.

REMEDY:

- The jaws, chin, teeth and all facial bone structure grows correctly and to its full potential, when Vitamin D is given in the form of Cod Liver Oil (in capsules) on a daily basis.
- Vitamin D is absolutely essential for Calcium to be absorbed in order to form healthy teeth and bones.

- Corrective surgery and steep medical expenses can be avoided with sufficient intake of Vitamin D. Braces and expensive dental care also become unnecessary with sufficient Vitamin D. These conditions are caused through a lack of this vitamin (providing adequate calcium and magnesium are taken).
- Bottle and pacifier use can deform jaws / airways.
- Breast suckling promotes good forward jaw growth and development.
- Bottle, pacifier and finger sucking put backward forces on the jaw during one of the most important periods of rapid forward growth.
- Dentists should advocate breastfeeding for about 6 to 12 months.

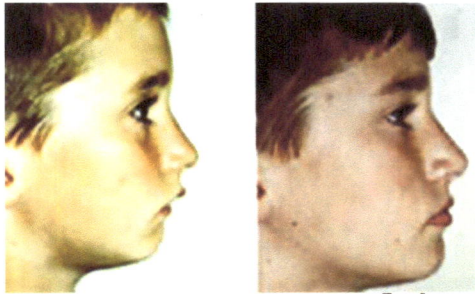

- Sixty percent of the face's growth occurs by age four.
- Research shows breast-fed infants have considerably less illness and fewer life-long health problems. Some of the health benefits of breastfeeding are due to better jaw and airway formation, although most credit has been given to the content of a nursing mother's milk.
- According to Van der Linden's Handbook of Facial Orthopedics—1982: Breastfeeding helps jaws and airways to develop properly.

IMMUNIZATIONS/Vaccines

The main focus of this book has been to share my own experiences with applied nutrition. However, with regard to vaccines, I have discovered disturbing evidence that compels me to reveal the risks. It is my responsibility to present other evidence and approaches. I will begin with my own testimony and what has worked for my family.

SYMPTOMS:

- Many infants and children suffer reactions to immunizations. Those symptoms can vary. It is common for a child to have a fever, a temperature and possibly some swelling and tenderness where the injection was given. Your baby could be quite miserable and grizzly as a result. In some cases very serious and life threatening reactions have occurred. However, both I and my family have avoided these by taking the following action.

REMEDY:

- *Before* the injection or medication is given, crush a 500 mg Vitamin C tablet (orange flavored), mix it into a thin paste with water and squirt this into the side of your baby's mouth with a syringe.

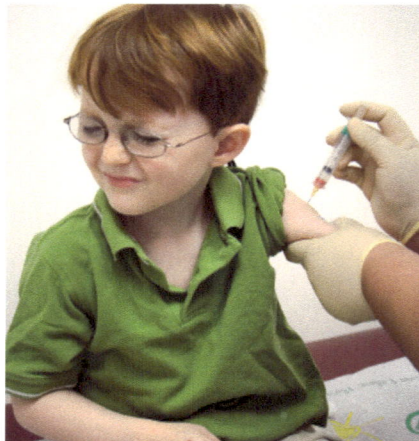

- *After* the injection, repeat this treatment with B5 (Pantothenic Acid) added to the Vitamin C in the same manner.

This can prevent adverse reactions to the medication altogether or minimize them. If your baby shows any sign that he is not his normal self, then give him a half dose every hour or two until bedtime. Treatment may be continued as required. If the symptoms do not show signs of reducing within 3–4 hours or if symptoms increase, consult your doctor.

- Vitamin C is a natural antibiotic, anti-histamine, anti-toxin and much more. According to Davis, when 500 mg to 1,000 mg of vitamin C are given with any medication, in any form, it is spent on reducing side affects from the medication in question. Vitamin C reduces the toxicity in drugs, and is claimed to enhance the effectiveness of a medication. This action has worked well for my family.
- Pantothenic Acid (Vitamin B5) supports the immune system in this situation and counteracts stress.

NOTE: My personal success with this protective measure, may have been enhanced by the high level of support given to my immune system (with supplements), which I have maintained over many years and extended to my children from infancy.

Regardless, it has proven to be effective for my children and grand children.

- With regard to Flu vaccines specifically, I prefer to rely on the protection of my own immune system, which I diligently supply with the nutrients it needs to do so—especially Vitamin D.
- The fact remains that vaccines can be life threatening. There is plenty of information available about this issue and I urge you to seek it and weigh the evidence before making the choice that you believe is best for you and your family.
- Do not blindly accept the propaganda promoted by Pharmaceutical companies.

The Dangers of Vaccines:

It is a documented fact that toxic chemicals have been found to be present in flu vaccines (and other medications).This is a huge controversial issue and I've received some strong opinions from those who are fore and against.

The (2009) H1N1 Swine Flu vaccine contains the adjuvant Squalene, which can trigger almost any auto immune disease known. It virtually sabotages and disables the body's natural immune system so that it undermines instead of protecting, the body's defences.

This is so important I seriously urge you to read it again.

The damage and suffering Squalene can do and has already caused, is staggering.

We can no longer accept on face value the assurances of the medical profession, (via pharmaceutical companies), that this vaccine is safe. It isn't. Infants have died from this.

It makes me wonder about other vaccines and other medications where I have seen side effects that are worse than the illness being treated.

As to the safety, the information has to originate from the manufacturer. Then this is passed onto the medical profession, who acts upon that information. And let's not forget there is a pre-existing connection, an established trust between drug companies and physicians which develops unconsciously during their training. The multimillion dollar drug companies help fund university courses in medicine and supply the course with the information about drugs. So it should come as no surprise that the medical profession should trust what ever the drug companies promote and act upon it.

I do *not* trust drug companies. They make their millions from our ill health and with the power that this money gives them they can do and say what ever they want. We only hear and see what they want us to hear and see.

They have the power to control and manipulate what the media says and what information they want revealed to us. They can block information they don't want us to know about to keep us dependent upon their products. They can foster fear and mistrust of any natural remedies that might succeed in threatening their profits. They can suppress or cover up nutritional breakthroughs, because they cannot patent them or make money from them. They can influence government policies and fund political campaigns.

And let's not forget; that statically thousands of people die each year from prescription drugs, as mentioned earlier. It's all about money and power.

The live viruses that are used in vaccines for the purpose of protection against disease (e.g. chicken pox, whooping cough, measles etc), rely on the human immune system to produce antibodies to protect individuals from a future attack of a specific disease. For the most part, this appears to work, but if your child happens to have a weak immune system at the time of injection it can reap distressing results.

Antibiotics which are commonly used through infancy and childhood have been known to cause diabetes in Infants as young as 18 months. Consider this issue carefully.

I am here to tell you that vitamins work better and without the risks or mortality rate.

JAUNDICE > see BILIRUBIN > Chapter 3

PARACETAMOL   P

- Speak to your doctor before administering pain relief,

such as Paracetamol, which should not be given to babies under three months of age.

- There is a danger of causing liver damage and kidney damage, especially in an infant where their organs are immature. Adults too are in the same danger if they exceed the recommended daily dose.
- Babies older than three months can be given Paracetamol or Calpol Infant Suspension.
- Be careful to follow instructions properly. Experts caution parents not to overdose their children and not to mix medications. Pick one and stick to it.
- Ensure your child drinks plenty of fluids and dress him/her in light, cool clothing.
- A tepid bath or sponging your baby with a cool wet cloth can also help reduce a high temperature.

REFLUX   R

SYMPTOMS:

- All babies bring up a little milk from time to time, but some regurgitate their food with great consistency. In the latter case, it might be reflux. Reflux is caused by an immature sphincter valve at the top of the stomach, which allows its contents to rise back up into the esophagus. This can cause a painful burning sensation for babies, as well as redecorating your furniture.

REMEDY:

- It is recommended that breast feeding mothers take a 1,000 IU Vitamin E supplement capsule daily, to strengthen the developing sphincter valve. However, if the mother is taking supplements with iron or food with added iron, Vitamin E needs to be taken 8 to 10 hours after the iron—iron cancels Vitamin E's ability to function if taken close together.

- For bottle-fed infants, try squeezing *½ a 500 IU Vitamin E capsule* directly into the baby's mouth twice a *day,* before feedings for 6–8 weeks. Then continue giving ½ to one *500 IU Vitamin E capsule* daily throughout childhood. Avoid formula that contains iron, try using goat's milk or full cream cow's milk when the Vitamin E is given. The Iron content renders Vitamin E totally ineffective.
- If you hold your baby in an upright position after feeding, for about twenty minutes, it can help—thanks to gravity alone. Feeding your baby less at each feeding but more frequently can also help.
- If your baby vomits constantly, more than five times daily, and is distressed after a feeding, visit your local doctor to see if there is a bigger issue than standard reflux.
- Constant throwing up after feedings means fewer nutrients are being absorbed and eventually your baby will become vulnerable to illness.

NOTE: I would try enzymes—as in the treatment for colic as soon as the reflux symptoms become a problem. The enzymes will help the digestive system and act as a temporary support. I would also give Vitamins B5 & C to support the immune system and to help compensate for the unknown amount of food/nutrients that are clearly not being processed effectively.

If this were my own child I would also squeeze half the contents of 500 IU capsule of Vitamin E into his mouth on a daily basis for one week then alternate days until the condition is corrected.

Follow the Supplement Guide No: 2 (refer page 30/31) for other nutrients required.

Note: If the vitamin E (oil) cannot be kept in the stomach,

then rub vitamin E oil into the skin of the buttocks and stomach daily. Cod Liver Oil can be applied in the same way. This method can sometimes be more efficient than taken orally as it reaches the blood stream without having to go through the digestive process. _Vitamin E helps repair & develop soft tissue—including the sphincter valve._ Supplements are essential to replace the food lost during this time. Other vitamins can also be absorbed through the Skin.

Cheryl Gi

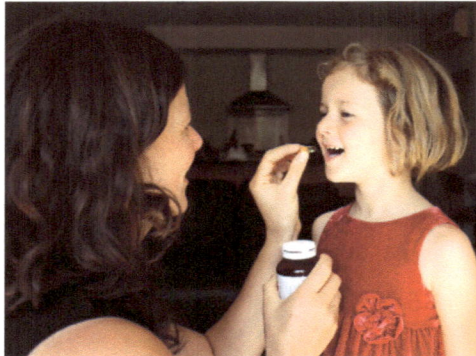

RESPIRATORY TRACT INFECTIONS   R

Respiratory tract infections are a sign of **Adrenal Exhaustion** and are covered in Chapter 3.

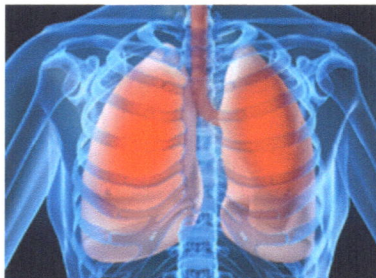

The 'Viruses & Infections' that follow; also refer to adrenal exhaustion and the immune system.

TEETHING   T

SYMPTOMS:

- Swollen gums, lots of drool, a change in sleeping patterns and feeding habits can all signal a tooth before the tooth becomes visible.
- Some mothers say their baby becomes cranky, runs a temperature, has unexplained diarrhea or develops a rash around their little mouth.

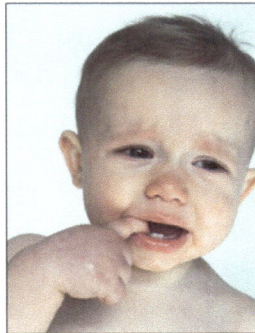

REMEDY:

- Teething can be painful and stressful for your baby. As soon as signs of teething appear, the following supplement works wonders: crush a 25mg tablet of Vitamin B5 with 250 mg of Vitamin C (orange flavored).
- Then mix these into a thin paste with a few drops of water and squeeze this into one side of your baby's mouth with a syringe. Supplement Guide No:2 is also recommended. If teething is causing severe distress the 'Natures Way' supplement—½ in the morning and at ½ night, with the extra doses of B5 and C above in between will make a huge difference. Supplements can also be mixed with fruit puree or jam.

- Do this morning and night for the entire teething period—when all teeth have surfaced. This will result in better sleep for baby (and parents) and support the immune system.
- Teething babies' inflamed gums can be soothed by having something cold or hard to bite on such as a teething ring. Try soaking a new flannel / face washing towel, in chamomile tea and then letting it cool in the fridge. Then give it to baby to suck on. Cold pureed food can help. If baby is in pain, a teething gel may offer some relief.
- Speak to your doctor before administering pain relief, such as Paracetamol, which should not be given to babies under three months of age. There is a danger of causing liver damage and kidney damage, especially in an infant where their organs are immature.

THRUSH

SYMPTOMS:

- Thrush is a severe rash that is the result of a fungus infection of *Candida albicans or Monilia albicans*. It is interesting to note that thrush can appear at either end of the digestive tract i.e. in the mouth or around the anal/genital area.
- Thrush appears when the intestinal bacteria fail to create B Vitamins and the healthy bacteria are in short supply. This means that a shortage of B Vitamins (a deficiency) is evident.
- A course of antibiotics will often trigger a thrush infection because the antibiotics upset the natural balance of 'good' & 'bad' bacteria in the bowel.
- Thrush is more likely to appear when there is a Vitamin A deficiency as well.

REMEDY:
- Thrush has been cleared up in 2 weeks or less when

100 mg of Niacinamide (one of the B vitamins) has been given each day to infants.

- Acidophilus culture or a tea spoon of yogurt added to expressed milk /formula will help restore the healthy balance of bacteria. Plain yoghurt can also be applied externally.
- A breastfeeding mother needs to rapidly increase the B Vitamins in her milk by increasing her intake of supplements.
- One high potency B complex capsule / tablet and at least 500 mg of Vitamin C, should be taken
- **morning and night** until the rash disappears. Continue a maintenance dose of B and C Vitamins once a day.
- Anti-fungal cream is available from the chemist to hasten the process. However, if B Vitamins are not restored to the body, the thrush will very likely re-occur.
- Alternatively, plain Yoghurt can be applied in the same way as an anti fungal cream, both internally (with an applicator for adult women) and externally.
- The thrush (candida) cannot thrive in the environment of healthy bacteria that yoghurt provides.
- The body has sent a clear message that it needs these nutrients —so give them, with supplements.

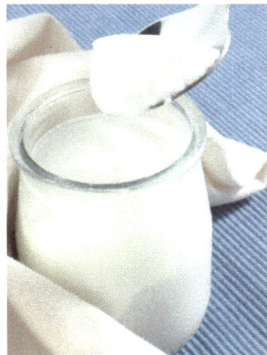

Yoghurt

VIRUSES AND INFECTIONS

FACTS:
- "Literally thousands of studies made the world over indicate that an infection simply cannot occur unless a weakness precedes it. Furthermore, the nutritional state at the time the infection sets in, determines the seriousness and duration of the illness and even whether a child survives."
- "If your baby's diet and intake of nutrients has been adequate, when bacteria or viruses gain entrance to his body, special lymph tissues produce protein substances known as antibodies. Each antibody "matches" a particular attacking virus or bacteria as a key does to a lock. These antibodies are his guardian angels, which render bacteria and viruses harmless and prevent infection from occurring."
- "Once specific antibodies have been created, your baby's lymph cells can reproduce them anytime they are needed, even years later, **provided his or her diet supplies the nutrients required to make them.**" Adelle Davis
- **A treatise on infections published by the World Health Organization states that Vitamin A deficiencies are present in almost every type of infection or infectious disease and it cites fifty scientific studies upon which this statement is based.**
- The human body is designed with marvelous defence systems to protect and maintain good health. It cannot do its job unless we supply it with the essential nutrients. Try running a car without oil in the engine or water in the radiator. Not good. It breaks down. In the same way our body will break down if we do not give it the quantities of nutrients it needs to function as it should.
- In the same way if we filled the gas tank of our car with contaminated gas or a weaker formula then the car would not function properly and in some cases may be dangerous. How many of us give more attention to our car than

we do to our own body? We need to make sure the nutrients and foods we put into our body are good quality.

- If grit or foreign bodies were to get into a car engine it would cause serious damage. In the same way, when chemicals from food, personal care products and our environment enter our body, they can and do serious damage over time. Antioxidants are vital in reversing this process.
- Adequate Vitamin A prevents infections in many ways. It protects the mucous membranes that cover **all** inside openings in the body, regardless. It protects every cell lining and prevents viruses or bacteria from entering.
- When we get an infection of this nature, it is an indication that we have not taken enough Vitamin A in conjunction with a full range of nutrients. Cod Liver Oil (capsules) are rich in Vitamin A and D.
- The body's need for all nutrients skyrockets for any illness. Dosages will vary between individuals—some need more of a specific vitamin(s) than others.

The Respiratory System

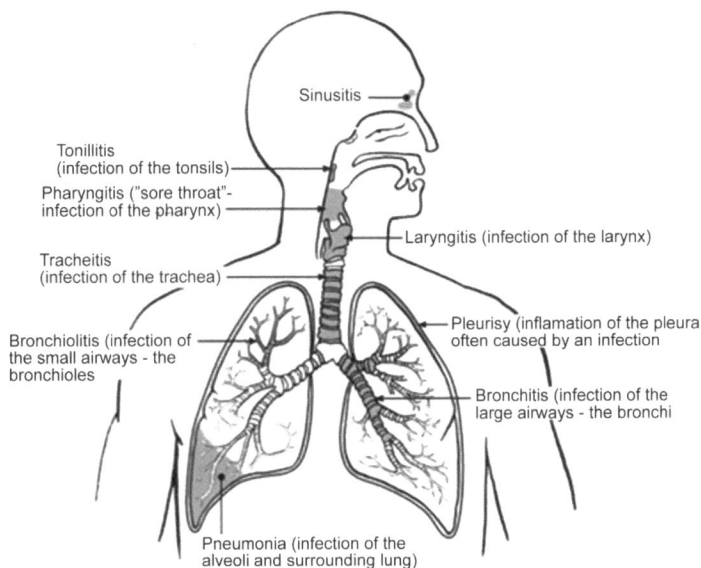

Infections of the respiratory tract

Author's note: Because of refined foods, nutrient poor foods due to soil deficiencies, etc, and our contaminated environment, it is not possible to supply the body with the amount of nutrients that it requires to maintain good health with food alone. Sadly, this situation is a fact of life now. The contributing factors are so long standing and so far reaching, the only feasible solution in the short term is to take supplements, educate yourself and again take supplements. Raise your children to understand and see this as being the norm and nothing out of the ordinary. It isn't difficult. Consume a variety of antioxidant foods and antioxidant supplements.

I take high potency Vitamins A, B, C, D & E, minerals and anti-oxidants daily. So too, my adult children and grand children take supplements. I can testify that during my 30 + years of remedial nutrition, my family's visits to the doctor were reduced by more than 40%.

Cheryl G.

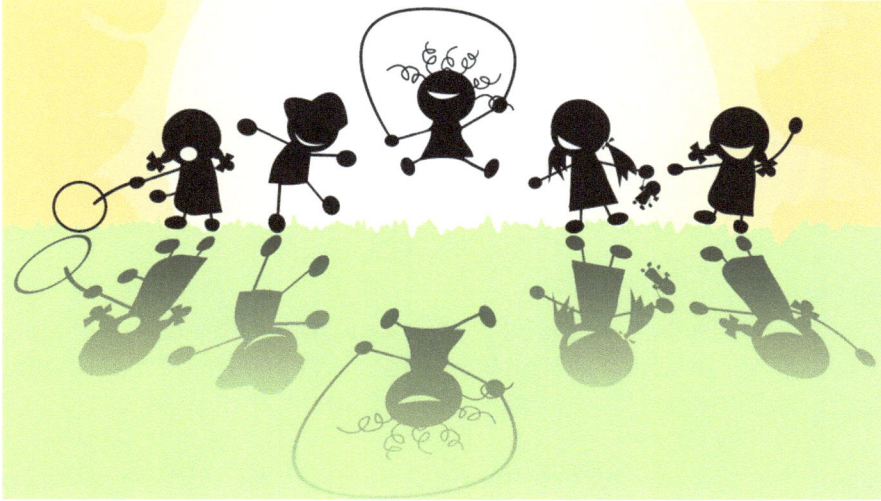

CHAPTER 6 – SUPPLEMENTS DURING PREGNANCY

Before we tackle a vitamin supplement regime, we need to combine it with a healthy diet, using the healthy diet pyramid as a guide.

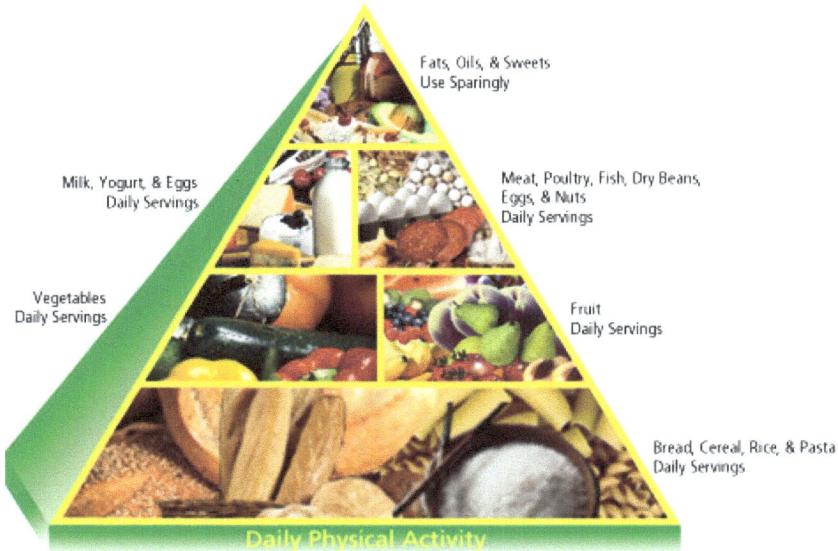

The advice that follows is a great starting point if you need to read up on good nutrition. For more information, ask your doctor to refer you to a dietician or visit the "Resources" section of www.help4healthykids.com you will find some healthy cookbooks among other topics.

Eat most:
Fruits, vegetables, seafood, legumes, grains, breads, cereals, rice and pasta which are all low in fat and provide energy-giving carbohydrate and a wide range of vitamins and minerals.

All of the previously mentioned, except fruits and vegetables are important sources of protein and all except seafood contain dietary fiber. Grains, breads, cereals, rice, pasta, legumes, vegetables and fruits are important sources of carbohydrate and energy.

Approximately 55%–60% of the total kilojoules we eat should come from carbohydrates, with complex carbohydrates supplying the most (40%–45%).

Eat Moderately:
Chicken, turkey, lean red meat, seafood, eggs, milk, cheese, yoghurt, nuts and seeds which are valuable for their protein, minerals and vitamins.

All except dairy products are good sources of Iron and Zinc, while dairy products are an excellent provider of Calcium. Each of these foods also supplies varying amounts of fats; however, their fats accompany other important dietary nutrients.

Eat Least:
Apart from some fats, such as olive oil, *most fats, sugars, white carbohydrates, salt and alcohol have little nutritional worth.*

Avoid:

Many processed and pre-prepared foods have a high fat and sugar content, as these are cheap filler ingredients. In small quantities these are not harmful, but in large quantities and over time, they can cause health problems.

Steps to a balanced diet:

Listed below are the National Health and Medical Research Council Recommendations which offer general guidelines for developing a balanced diet:

1. Enjoy a wide variety of nutritious foods
2. Eat plenty of breads and cereals (preferably whole grain), vegetables, legumes and fruits
3. Eat a diet low in fat, particularly saturated fat.
4. Maintain a healthy body weight by balancing physical activity and food intake
5. Eat only a moderate amount of sugars and foods containing added sugars
6. Choose low salt foods and use salt sparingly
7. Encourage and support breastfeeding
8. Eat foods containing Calcium. This is particularly important for girls and women.
9. Eat foods containing Iron.

Healthy foods for pregnant women:

It is important to choose a wide variety of foods to ensure the nutritional needs of both mother and baby are met. Try to eat:

- Lots of fruit and vegetables, whole grain breads and cereals
- Moderate amounts of low fat dairy foods and lean meats
- Limited amounts of foods high in fat, sugar and salt
- Lean meat, chicken and fish
- Dried beans and lentils
- Nuts and seeds
- Low fat milk, cheese and yoghurt
- Green leafy vegetables

Folic Acid (Folate)

Folate (known as Folic Acid when added to foods) is a B-group vitamin found in a variety of foods. Some breakfast cereals, breads and juices are fortified with Folic Acid. This will be listed on the nutrition label of these products.

As well as a healthy diet, it is also recommended that a Folic Acid supplement be taken prior to conception and for the first three months of pregnancy, to reduce the risk of neural tube defects such as spina bifida. Folate taken over this period can prevent up to 7 out of 10 cases of neural tube defects.

If you are planning a pregnancy or are in the early stages of pregnancy, you should increase your Folate intake by an additional 0.4 mg (400 mcg) per day above the recommended daily intake (RDI) of 0.6 mg (600 mcg) per day for pregnancy. That is 1000 micrograms per day.

Excellent sources of folate include:

Very Good sources include:	Others:
• Asparagus	Hazelnuts
• Cabbage	Vegemite
• Bran flakes	Leeks
• Cauliflower	Oranges
• Broccoli	Orange juice
• Parsnip	Salmon
• Brussels sprouts	Potatoes
• Dried beans	Tomatoes
• Parsley	Peas
• Liver	Walnuts
• Chickpeas / Lentils	Peanuts
• Spinach.	Wheat germ

Iron
Pregnancy increases the need for Iron in the diet. Leafy greens like silver beet are a good source.

Pregnancy in adolescence
- Pregnant adolescents need more nutrients than adult women, because they are still growing. Adolescents may give birth to smaller infants because they are competing with the growing fetus for nutrients
- Anemia is more common among adolescents than older women. Calcium intake is also important because young women have not yet reached their peak bone mass and inadequate Calcium intake may increase the risk of osteoporosis developing later in life.

Nausea and vomiting
Nausea and vomiting, especially 'morning sickness,' are common during pregnancy – particularly in the first trimester.
- Small carbohydrate snacks (a sandwich or fruit) every two to three hours may provide some relief during the day.
- Try a light snack e.g. cheese on dry biscuits just before bed PLUS a 50 mg Vitamin B6 tablet. A B6 *deficiency* can cause morning sickness.
- The following suggestions may also help:
- Eat some dry bread, biscuits or cereal before getting up in the morning. Get up slowly, avoiding sudden movements.
- Drink liquids between, rather than with, meals to avoid bloating, which can trigger vomiting.
- Avoid large meals and greasy, highly spiced foods. It may be better to have 6 small meals and/or graze throughout the day.
- Suck something sour like a lemon.
- Relax rest and get fresh air as much as possible. Keep rooms well ventilated and odour free.
- Slowly sip an effervescent drink (specifically for upset stomachs), when you feel nauseated.

- Try food and drinks containing ginger as these sometimes relieve nausea.

Heartburn

Heartburn is common in pregnancy; partly due to the pressure on the abdomen as the baby grows. If like me you experience heartburn with no discomfort apart from burping occasionally, (starting 3 weeks after conception), you may escape morning sickness completely as I did.

Things to avoid

Alcohol during pregnancy

Consuming alcohol during pregnancy increases the risk of a miscarriage, low birth weight, congenital deformities and effects on the baby's intelligence.

Some foods are more prone to contamination than others. Avoid these foods in your diet if you are pregnant:
- Soft cheeses, such as brie, camembert and ricotta – these are safe only if served cooked and hot.
- Pre-cooked or pre-prepared cold foods that will not be reheated – for example, pre-prepared salads, pate, quiches and delicatessen meats like ham and salami.
- Raw seafood such as oysters and sashimi or smoked seafood such as salmon (canned varieties are safe)
- Non-pasteurized foods
- Soft-serve ice cream

The organism that causes listeria is destroyed by heat, so properly cooked foods are not a risk.

Salmonella

Salmonella is a cause of food poisoning that can trigger a miscarriage. The most likely sources of salmonella are raw eggs and under-cooked meat and poultry.

Good food hygiene

Good food hygiene is the best way to reduce the risk of salmonella and listeria infections. Suggestions include:

- Always wash your hands before and after preparing food
- Keep your kitchen surfaces clean
- Do not let uncooked food contaminate cooked food.
- Wash fruit, vegetables and salad before eating.
- Cook food thoroughly.
- Keep pets away from kitchen surfaces.
- Wear rubber gloves when handling cat litter trays or gardening.
- Store food at correct temperatures.

Mercury in fish

It is suggested that pregnant women eat 2–3 servings of fish every week for good health. Caution should be exercised when choosing the type of fish you will eat.

There are a few types of fish that need to be limited because they contain high levels of mercury, which is dangerous for the developing fetus. These are: swordfish, broadbill, marlin and shark (flake) – limit to 1 serve per fortnight, deep-sea perch, 1 serve per week.

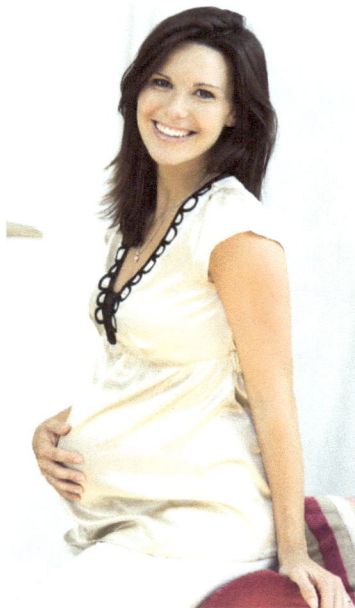

Antioxidant Foods:
- water, green tea, grape seed extract
- avocado, broccoli, onions, peppers, soy, spinach, and sprouts, hot peppers, leeks, daikon radishes
- açai berries, goji berries, apples, blueberries, pomegranates, pumpkin, kiwi, oranges, tomatoes
- wild salmon, turkey, eggs
- beans, barley, seeds, nuts, lentils, oats, walnuts and buckwheat
- cinnamon, dark chocolates, garlic, honey, extra virgin olive oil ("cold pressed"), sea salt, natural yogurt & kefir
- sea vegetables, irish moss, umeboshi plums, wheat grass, miso

Now that we know how to achieve a healthy-as-possible diet, it's important to understand why you need to work towards maintaining it throughout pregnancy, coupled with your supplements.

Inadequate food intake can have serious consequences for your baby. Malnutrition can retard the growth of the placenta and may increase the risk of a miscarriage and a premature or low birth weight baby. (Refer to my story in chapter two). These babies are more vulnerable at birth and throughout life.

A severely malnourished mother may prevent optimal brain function in her baby, as the most rapid brain development occurs in the last trimester of pregnancy and in the baby's first month.

It is important to note that when malnourished, the fetus will divert whatever is available *to* the cells that need it immediately and *away from* those cells that aren't important <u>until later in life.</u>

This means <u>in</u>adequate nutrition during pregnancy can continue to affect your child later in life and may contrib-

ute to middle-aged diseases such as high blood pressure, coronary artery disease and obesity.

A well nourished mother is more likely to produce a good sized baby that is active and more mentally alert, and less likely to suffer from colic, diarrhea, anemia or infection.

Supplements during Pregnancy and Breast feeding

The following is the Daily supplement regime I followed during pregnancy and breast feeding:

- 1 high dosage B complex tablet morning and night. If the brand you choose has less than 400 mcg of Folic Acid (Folate), then extra will have to be taken. The minimum is about 400 mcg daily.
- A woman cannot get enough B vitamins during pregnancy. (You can drop to one per day during breast feeding, but if problems arise with not enough breast milk, then return to 2 per day and drink plenty of water.)
- One 500 IU of natural Vitamin E (capsule) daily and apply Vitamin E oil (from capsules) to the stomach to reduce/avoid stretch marks. Can also be applied to the mouth of the birth canal to increase elasticity and minimize the need for stitches.
- Two Cod Liver Oil capsules daily for Vitamin A and D.
- 1000 mg Vitamin C per day. Start off with 500 mg for 3 days then gradually increase to 1000 mg.
- 2 Calcium with Magnesium tablets at bedtime.
- One Liver capsule or tablet daily for natural Iron intake for first 6 months. (The ferrous form of Iron tends to cause constipation)
- One multi-mineral supplement alternate days for the first 6 months then daily.
- Once per week I had 2 drops of Lugol's solution (Iodine from chemist) in fruit juice/water during the second trimester for thyroid health. I applied Zinc cream to one arm pit (once per week) at night for my intake

of Zinc.

- **During times of stress or threatened illness, I increased my B5 and Vitamin C intake. I also made pep-up drink by vitamizing 2 cups of whole, organic, non-homogenized milk, 1 egg, 1 banana, 2 tablespoons of plain yogurt and 2 drops of vanilla essence. Home made yogurt is best as it is not tart (sour). ½ a teaspoon of honey may be added. I would sip this between meals. This is also good if for any reason you skip a meal.**

- While breast feeding I took the supplements above, plus Calcium and Potassium.

- It is a good idea to commence supplements *before conception* especially if you have been taking oral contraceptives (or injections). Contraceptives of this nature destroy the B Vitamins and Vitamin E, which emphasizes and increases the need for these to be supplemented.

- Smoking robs both you and the baby of much needed vitamins and lays a foundation for an underweight baby who is likely to suffer bouts of sickness more often, than one whose mother is a non-smoker.

A mother to be who has made it her business to be nutritionally aware and to work with an obstetrician who is also nutritionally oriented, will be more likely to recognize any sign of a deficiency and be able to correct it.

However, no doctor can do your eating for you. *You* are responsible for your health and the health of your baby.

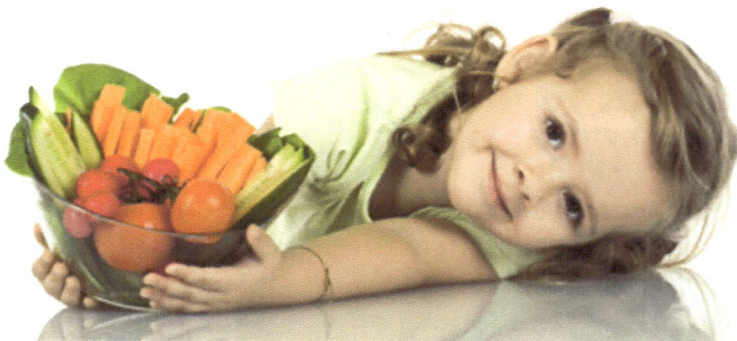

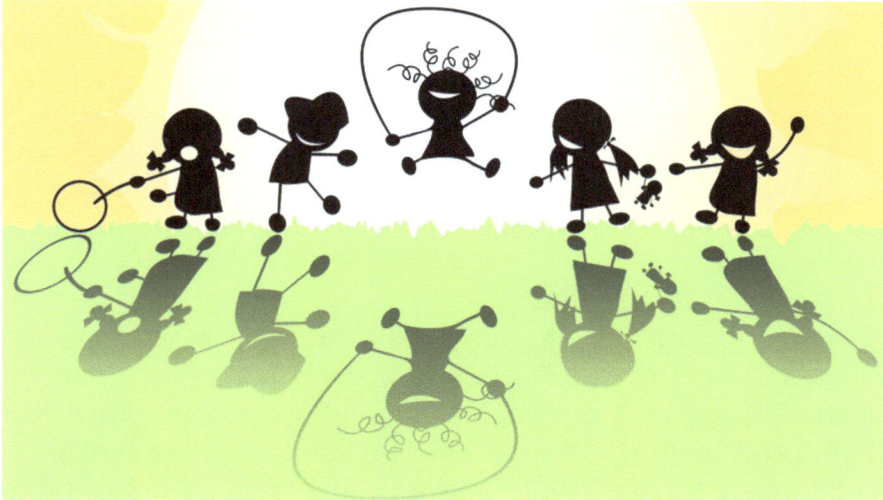

CHAPTER 7 – WHAT TO DO WHEN THINGS GO WRONG

It is fair to say that women expect and/or hope that their pregnancy will all be smooth sailing. All too often however, there are conditions that arise that can be unhealthy for both mother and the unborn infant. Some of those conditions can be life-threatening. Below are some of those unwelcome and unanticipated conditions and what you can do about them.

BREAST FEEDING and Sore Nipples

Breast feeding your infant has so many benefits that can have a life long impact on his/her health. I breast fed my three children 18 months each. Even when working part time (5 hours per day) I managed to continue breast feeding.

I simply gave my 6 month old daughter a 'top up' feed about ½ an hour before leaving for work, regardless of the previous feeding time, and then again when I returned home. I had small portions of fruit puree and yoghurt available, as well as expressed milk, in case she became hungry while I was away. At work, if my breasts became too full I simply went to the restroom and expressed a little milk to reduce the pressure. My milk production adjusted naturally within 2 weeks so that I no longer had to express milk.

To prevent **sore nipples,** you need to begin massaging the nipples 3–4 months BEFORE your baby is born. From an outer circumference of 3 centimeters around the nipple, draw your thumb and fingers from separate directions towards the nipples. Then gently roll the nipple between. Use vitamin E oil from a capsule to lubricate this action. This method toughens the nipples so they do not become sore. It also stimulates colostrum and early milk production.

If this method has been previously overlooked and soreness occurs, still apply the preventive action between feeds; using less pressure according to your comfort zone.

BLOOD PRESSURE (Hypertension)

Blood pressure exists when the heart's pumping pushes the blood against the walls of the blood vessels. The magnitude of blood pressure is determined by the amount of blood being pumped out of the heart per beat (the stroke volume) and the resistance encountered as it passes through the blood vessels (peripheral resistance).

During pregnancy the risk of high blood pressure (HBP) increases simply because the heart is now responsible for taking care of two bodies – yours and your baby's.

High blood pressure is when the actual force of the blood flow places too much pressure against the walls of blood vessels.

SYMPTOMS:

- There are often no obvious signs of high blood pressure. The safest action is to have your physician regularly check for this condition throughout pregnancy. If this condition is present and left untreated it can lead to complications and serious health risks to the mother and her baby. (See Edema→Toxemia/Eclampsia).

REMEDY:

- High potency supplements, especially B complex, throughout pregnancy are a prerequisite.
- Avoid over exertion, heavy lifting, becoming over weight. Extra weight has a direct link to HBP.
- Gentle exercise is fine. The diet recommendations in Chapter 6 will assist.
- Avoid emotional stress/stressful encounters as much as possible.
- Lycopene—a natural substance in tomatoes has been found to reduce high blood pressure (HBP).
- Studies conducted, (Steven K. Clinton, M.D., Ph.D.) suggest that consuming tomato products is more effective than Lycopene in supplement form.
- Lycopene is also present in watermelon, papaya, pink grapefruit and guava.
- Keep taking high potency B vitamins – Choline (one of the B complex vitamins) has been given to people with dangerously high blood pressure, resulting in blood pressure returning to normal.

EDEMA

SYMPTOMS:

- Edema is the retention of fluids in the tissues and is often evidenced in the form of puffy fingers and swollen feet/

ankles. This condition should not be perceived as trivial—it can become a serious condition (Eclampsia) if it is not addressed straight away. Eclampsia can be life threatening.

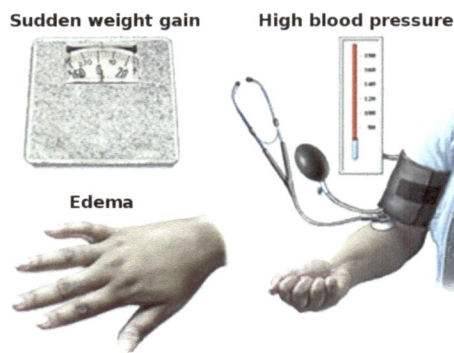

- Edema caused by Vitamin B6 deficiency: Regardless of how much protein is eaten, the body proteins cannot be utilized unless B6 is in plentiful supply. Therefore, a lack of B6 has the same effect as not eating enough protein.
- The liver can no longer process albumin, which interferes with the collection of urine and causes waste laden fluids to be left in the tissues.
- The lack of any nutrient that impacts on the production of albumin or causes it to be lost through urine or the bowel can cause edema.
- Stress is another cause that needs to be watched. It is an outside factor that causes the body to use up valuable nutrients in its effort to neutralize that stress. For example, an emotional upset can result in swollen feet and fingers within 24 hours.
- For the body, pregnancy is a form of stress in itself.

REMEDY:

- An extra 50 mg of B6 with each meal for 4 days and an increase in B5 coupled with Vitamin C to counter the stress is recommended. If swelling reoccurs, then take extra B complex daily and B6 as required until the baby is born.

- This is on top of the supplement regime you are already following. (Note: If you use my supplement regime in Chapter 6, it can prevent this condition.)
- <u>Remember, when any illness arises, it is a signal that your body needs more nutrients.</u>

-

LABOR AND DELIVERY

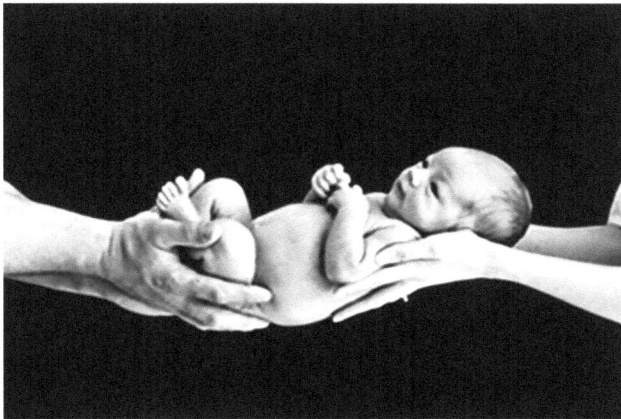

SYMPTOMS:

- A long and pain-filled labor can be exhausting.
- Weak muscles make the labor longer and more difficult.
- Not enough elasticity in the vaginal tissues can cause tearing or make it necessary for the doctor to perform an episiotomy. This involves a cut at the vaginal entrance and stitches after the baby is born.

REMEDY:

- Calcium has been known to decrease muscular pain. If 2000 mg of Calcium is taken between the time labor first starts and the time you arrive at the hospital it has been known to noticeably reduce the pain.

- Of course Vitamin D and Magnesium are required to ensure total absorption of the Calcium.
- Zinc promotes a quicker and easier delivery. Apply Zinc cream to an arm pit for two nights before the delivery date and again at the onset of labor. Or take it in tablet form if you prefer.
- Vitamin E (Alpha Tocopherol Acetate) and adequate protein promote strong muscles. Muscles become extremely weak if Vitamin E is deficient.
- Vitamin E should be taken 10 hours after Iron salts. Inorganic Iron neutralizes Vitamin E if the two of them meet in the digestive tract.
- Vitamin E also increases the elasticity of the vaginal tissues. 1000 IU of Vitamin E shortly before leaving home to go to the hospital tremendously increases the expandability of the vaginal area.
- Certain hormones cause this unusual elasticity to occur towards a full term pregnancy, but only when Vitamin E is adequate.
- Vitamin C also assists in keeping elasticity in the vaginal tissues and tearing can occur if there is a lack of this nutrient.
- Dr. Fred Klenner, (formerly chief of staff at the Memorial Hospital, Reidsville, North Carolina), **recommended that all pregnant women under his care take up to 10,000 mg of Vitamin C daily.** NB: It is best to start with 500 mg of Vitamin C and slowly increase the dosage week by week, as the body needs time to adjust to high dosages. A sudden increase in high dosages of Vit. C may cause loose bowel movements.
- This high quantity was found to result in easy deliveries and that hemorrhaging, anemia and stretch marks were greatly reduced.
- The need for vitamin B5 (Pantothenic Acid), is enormous just before birth, perhaps because it is the anti stress vitamin. And it is fare to say that both Mother and baby experience stress during the birthing process.

MASTITIS

SYMPTOMS:

- Mastitis is a very painful breast infection, which can occur in the first few weeks of breast-feeding.
- Bacteria gets into the milk ducts and the breast becomes hard, red and inflamed.
- This is not to be confused with engorged breasts which generally occur in the first days of milk production. This is addressed early, by massaging the milk ducts from the outer breast towards the nipples to express the build up of milk. (I had an experienced nurse who was kind enough to help me).

REMEDY:

- Antibiotics are usually prescribed by a physician to help clear up the infection. This condition needs to be checked by a doctor.
- Use warm water on the infected area of the breast before breast-feeding to help stimulate letdown (the milk ejection reflex).
- Breast-feed or express milk frequently, using both breasts. Lactation consultants recommend first breast-feeding from the unaffected breast until let-down (milk ejection reflex) occurs and then switch to the breast with mastitis.
- Breast-feed only until the breast is soft.
- Apply icy compresses to the breasts after breast-feeding to relieve pain and swelling.
- Drink fluids and get enough rest.
- Ask a physician about whether over-the-counter pain relievers are safe to use before taking any.
- I would increase Vitamin # (1000 IU) and C (1000 mg to 5000 mg for anti inflammatory action and anti biotic action,) until the symptoms are significantly reduced.
- Continue your normal supplement routine for all required

nutrients and increase vitamin B5 to counter-act the stress.

- Once full recovery has been achieved, remain on a supplement dose that meets the demands of breast feeding.
- If the stress of this condition causes reduced milk production, persevere with frequent feeding, continue supplements and believe in yourself.

MORNING SICKNESS / NAUSEA

SYMPTOMS:

- Generally, an unpleasant upheaval of the stomach's contents when you get up in the morning. Nausea and vomiting are common during pregnancy—particularly in the first trimester.
- For some women, it doesn't end there. They continue to vomit throughout the day. Sometimes it can be triggered by the smell of food.

REMEDY:

- Small snacks may provide some relief during the day.
- Try a light snack e.g. cheese (avoiding soft cheese) on dry biscuits just before bed, PLUS a 50 mg Vitamin B6 tablet. A B6 *deficiency* contributes to morning sickness.
- Some doctors give B6 injections to alleviate this condition depending upon how severe it is.
- Ensure ALL vitamin supplements are taken to compensate during this crucial time of the development in the first three months. Take supplements with food—not on an empty stomach.
- The following actions may ease the condition:
- Eat some dry bread, biscuits or cereal before getting up in the morning. Get up slowly, avoiding sudden movements. Drink liquids between, rather than with, meals to avoid bloating, which can trigger vomiting.

- It may be better to have 6 small meals and/or graze throughout the day. Avoid large meals and greasy, highly spiced foods.
- Suck something sour like a lemon.
- Relax rest and get fresh air as much as possible. Keep rooms well ventilated and odor free.

MISCARRIAGE

SYMPTOMS:

- Every nutrient plays a role in helping you carry your baby through a normal pregnancy.
- When these nutrients are lacking in any way, it leaves a woman vulnerable towards a miscarriage.
- There may be any number of surface triggers for a miscarriage to occur e.g. sickness, over doing activities or stressful situations. But the foundational cause is more likely to be a pre existing deficiency.
- Oral antibiotics taken during the first 3 months can also cause a miscarriage.
-

REMEDY:

- Prepare your body before conception by starting a supplement regime.
- Have your partner participate in this regime.
- **Vitamin E** is necessary for the division of cells and it works with Vitamin A to create a healthy uterine lining for the newly fertilized egg.
- **Folic Acid** has a very important function, it forms the nucleic acids DNA and RNA, which carry hereditary patterns and help synthesize the protein in every cell of the body from the moment of conception.
- An example of my own supplement regime is found in Chapter 6, to act as a guide.
- Continue to supplement and eat wisely.

- Eat several small meals throughout the day rather than three big meals.

PREMATURE DELIVERIES

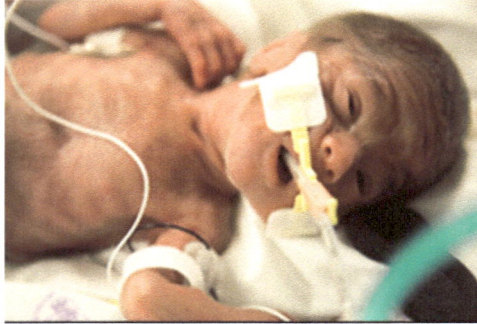

SYMPTOMS:

- Premature birth makes a baby more vulnerable to all kinds of illnesses.
- Because hormones that are released late in pregnancy cause the vaginal membranes to be more elastic, any birth that occurs before these hormones are produced is usually a difficult one.
- Prolonged nursery care in an incubator is not only expensive, but it complicates the breast feeding process at a time when an infant desperately needs it.
- During the final few weeks of pregnancy significant brain development occurs, but this is not permitted with a premature birth.

REMEDY:

- The best 'cure' is to prevent this situation.
- Premature birth means that an infant's lungs, other organs and muscles have not fully developed and can cause other problems. E.g. Not enough strength to en-

able the sucking motion for breast feeding. Severe jaundice may develop.

- General health is very fragile and vulnerable.
- It can be avoided by following a particularly healthy diet (discussed earlier) and an effective supplement regime like the one in Chapter 6.
- If a premature birth occurs, an immediate supplement regime is recommended and every effort made to provide your baby with your 'supplemented' breast milk. This means a full range of high potency vitamins is to be taken immediately to 1) to provide quality breast milk to your baby and 2) to correct the deficiencies that caused the condition from the beginning.
- Personally, as soon as my baby came home from hospital I would begin supplements for him/her to compensate for being 'short changed' in this way. (Refer to Chapter 3)

STRETCH MARKS

SYMPTOMS:

- Stretch marks are formed when skin has lost its ability to stretch further and so it 'tears' without becoming detached.
- These tend to form on the stomach, hips and breasts.

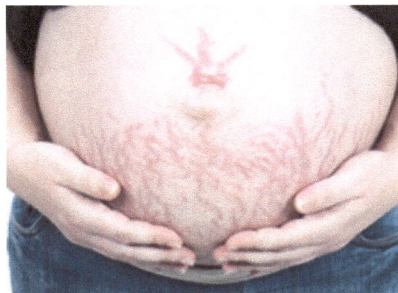

REMEDY:

- The condition of your skin and general health before pregnancy will have an impact on how well the condition responds to treatment, especially if you have been taking oral contraceptives prior to conception.
- However, an inclusion of Vitamin E and A (in Cod Liver Oil capsules) with a high dosage supplement regime during pregnancy, plus a daily massage ofVitamin E oil onto the areas concerned will minimize or prevent stretch marks.
- Vitamin E has amazing healing powers with soft tissues when combined with all other nutrients and adequate protein intake.
- If some stretch marks still manage to show, continue with the Vitamin E orally and externally until they fade away. Sometimes a few months of nutritional remedies cannot make up for a lifetime of neglect, but they can improve the situation.
- High dosages of Vitamin C also assist in preventing stretch marks (page 98).

TOXEMIA or ECLAMPSIA

SYMPTOMS:

- Toxemia is a serious condition that can be fatal if left untreated.
- High to very high blood pressure, that may cause dizziness, headaches, ringing in the ears and sometimes hemorrhages in the eyes. The elevated blood pressure may represent a serious health hazard.
- High blood pressure, edema, albumin in the urine, and kidney damage are all symptoms of toxemia.

REMEDY:

- Toxemia needs to be monitored/treated by a doctor.

- Choline (one of the B complex vitamins) has been given to people with dangerously high blood pressure, resulting in blood pressure returning to normal, edema to be corrected and albumen to disappear in urine.
- It is important to note however, that a person or child who is deficient in one vitamin is generally deficient in many. If the Toxemia symptoms materialize, take 5–6 high potency B Complex vitamin tablets (or capsules) throughout each day (e.g. every 2 hours) until the symptoms disappear. Then revert to 1 tablet with each meal.
- This condition can be prevented by following a healthy diet (discussed earlier) and an effective supplement regime like the one in Chapter 6.

VARICOSE VEINS

SYMPTOMS:

- More than one tenth of all pregnant women suffer with varicose veins before the birth of their first babies.
- The medical opinion is that varicose veins are caused by defective valves and are complicated by the pressure of the enlarged uterus on the veins of the abdomen.
- Scientists have shown that varicose veins occur when a clot forms in the vein and blocks the passage of blood. Generally the clot attaches itself to the blood vessel wall causing it to become irritated, swollen, and inflamed. This combination of symptoms completely blocks the vein so that no blood can pass through; resulting in ugly aching legs.

REMEDY:

- Very effective results have been attained with high doses of Vitamin E.
- Vitamin E has a role in maintaining the integrity of cells and all soft tissues in the body.

- When cells breakdown, they form a clot. This 'break-down' can be prevented by taking Vitamin E. (500 IU or more).
- 1,000 mg of Vitamin C daily also hastens recovery.
- To prevent varicose veins, stick to an excellent diet and a supplement regime similar to the one in chapter 6. Monitor the condition of your leg veins. If they begin to ache and swell a little, immediately increase Vitamin E & C on top of the existing supplements consumed and continue this as long as necessary.
- Hemorrhoids are a form of varicose veins in the bowel.
- Applying Aloe Vera pulp directly from the plant to the affected area will give quick relief from the pain of hemorrhoids. (A combination of all the previous 'dot' points will be the most effective.)
- During labor and the 'bearing down' process the pressure can exacerbate hemorrhoid problems but recovery is quick once the baby is born.

General Well-Being Tips

Tiredness:
Do not push yourself too hard to get your house work done or your list of tasks for the day. Have frequent rests when you feel tired. Pace yourself, prioritize and nibble at these tasks through out each day. Don't be afraid to ask for help if you need it and don't stress.

Try a freshly juiced fruit and vegetable drink combination for a pick-me-up.

Back ache:
Avoid bending over the sink (to do the dishes etc) for prolonged periods, especially during the last two months when you feel like a beached whale. If you don't have a dish washer, soak all the dirty dishes in a sink of hot soapy water for 30 minutes and then rinse them. Only scrub the items that need it.

Warm a 'wheat bag' in the microwave for 2 minutes, wrap it in a scarf or cloth and apply it to the area of the back that is aching. Lay down like this for 20 to 30 minutes. A 'wheat bag' is simply a long rectangular bag about 10 centimeters x 30 centimeters; filled with grains of wheat. This works wonders.

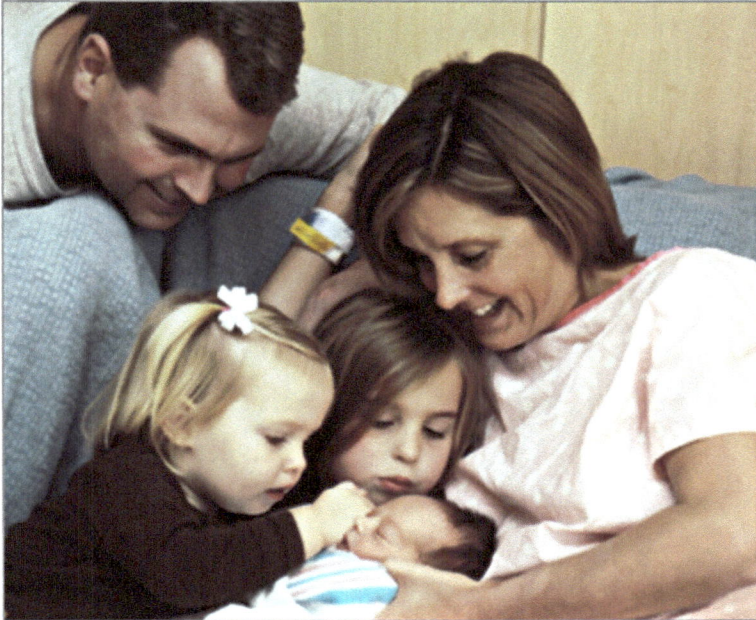

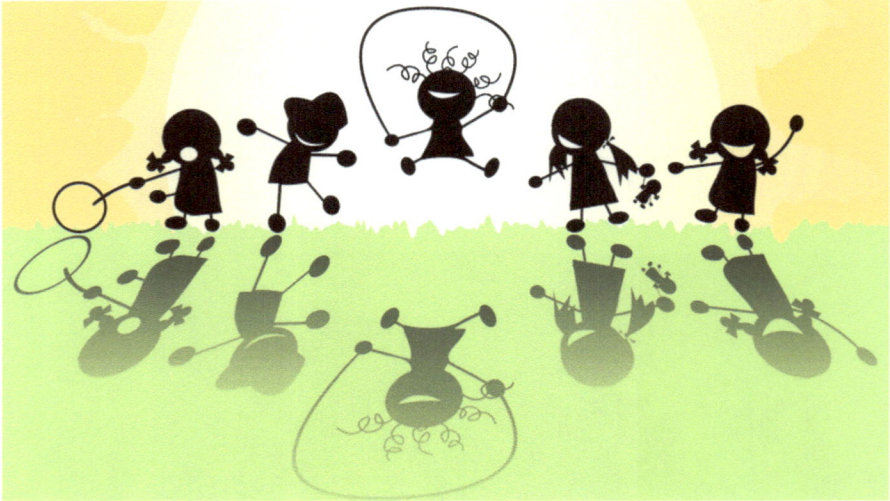

CHAPTER 8 – TWO AMAZING VITAMINS

VITAMIN E

Vitamin E is the most neglected and under-rated vitamin. This vitamin alone can prevent untold suffering in terms of health.

- Blood analyses have shown that all newborn infants are low in Vitamin E. Hemolytic anemia can occur as the essential fatty acids in the walls of red blood cells are exposed to larger amounts of oxygen than cells in other parts of the body and they break down to such an extent that this form of anemia can occur. Premature babies are especially vulnerable. This type of anemia cannot be prevented or corrected by any other nutrient.
- If you are not breast feeding, be sure that the formula provides 400 IU per day. If it does not then a supplement

is required. As mentions in chapter 4, jaundice also occurs when Vitamin E is not supplied.

- Lack of this vitamin can also cause brain damage. A short supply of red blood cells as described above creates oxygen starvation, as the red blood cells are needed to supply oxygen to the brain. A lack of oxygen can cause mental retardation.

- Vitamin E used to be generously supplied by foods and was obtained from unrefined breads and cereals and all natural sources of vegetable oils. Once grains are milled and oils are refined in our over-processed food supply, Vitamin E is lost. The introduction of skim milk has also impacted on the lack of this vitamin, as it prevents absorption and the transportation of Vitamin E in the blood.

- Like all the fat-soluble vitamins: Vitamin (A, D, E and K), Vitamin E is carried across the intestinal wall by being combined with an ingredient of bile, which is present in the small intestine *only after fat has been eaten*.

- See how just a minor thing like skim milk or fat-reduced milk can affect the way our body functions? Everything we do or don't do has consequences, everything we eat or don't eat, has an effect for good or bad on our health. This is why it is so important to eat a broad range of quality foods, and to stick to a high-potency supplement regime. The supplements act as a safety net for the nutrients and/or foods that *may* be missing from your diet. I say *"may"* to be polite—the reality is nutrients **are** missing.

- Fortunately for breast-fed babies, if a mother's diet is high in quality and a supplement regime is followed, the amount of Vitamin E for an infant remains high. In fact, colostrum, which is the first milk secreted, is seven times richer in this vitamin than in the milk that follows.

- When buying this vitamin, look for **d-alpha tocopherol acetate** on the label. This is the most effective in its natural form as opposed to the synthetic Vitamin E. In its natural form Vitamin E is non-toxic.

- When oil or polyunsaturated fats are eaten, they

increase the need for Vitamin E by anywhere up to 400%.

- One of the first problems to arise when Vitamin E is under supplied is that cells break down throughout the whole body and weaken the muscles. Gradually, the destroyed muscle cells are replaced by inert scar tissue. When so much destruction has occurred that muscles can no longer function, the condition can be diagnosed as muscular dystrophy.
- Illnesses related to Vitamin E deficiencies have become progressively more serious as this nutrient has been ignored or destroyed during food processing. A review of illnesses associated with these deficiencies during pregnancy, reveals a risk of miscarriages, varicose veins, phlebitis, pulmonary embolisms, premature births, still births, malformed or mentally retarded children and anemia.
- Vitamin E is an anti-oxidant which intercepts free radicals and therefore prevents lipid destruction chain reactions. It maintains the integrity of cell membranes.
- Vitamin E is essential for the maintenance of the heart function, the functioning of sexual organs and for cell protection. It is part of the immune system and protects us from skin and scar tissue and inflammation.
- A vitamin E deficiency is hard to recognize as it has no visible indication. It may result in impaired balance and coordination or muscle weakness.
- Because α-tocopherol has the ability to enhance antibody formation **extra Vitamin E needs to be taken by people suffering from the flu or other viruses.**
- Even though its name makes it sound like a single substance, Vitamin E is actually a family of fat-soluble vitamins that are active throughout the body. Some members of the Vitamin E family are called tocopherols. These members include alpha tocopherol, beta tocopherol, gamma tocopherol, and delta tocopherol.
- Although we humans must breathe oxygen to stay alive,

oxygen is a risky substance inside the body because it can make molecules overly react. When oxygen-containing molecules become too reactive, they can start damaging the cell structures around them. **Vitamin E helps prevent the condition known as oxidative stress.**

- Vitamin E directly protects the skin from ultraviolet radiation. In numerous research studies, Vitamin E applied topically to the skin has been shown to prevent UV damage. When the diet contains Vitamin E rich foods, or supplements, Vitamin E can travel to the skin cell membranes and exert this same protective effect.

- The transfer of chemical information from one cell to another, or across different structures inside of a cell is referred to as cell signaling. Many researchers believe that the cell signaling cannot be facilitated without the help of Vitamin E.

- In many research studies, low levels of Vitamin E are associated with digestive system problems where nutrients are poorly absorbed from the digestive tract. These problems include pancreatic disease, gallbladder disease, liver disease, and celiac disease.

- Because unseen scar tissue e.g. ear infections, rheumatic fever, can interfere with body function, **Vitamin E intake should be increased during all illnesses**, before and after surgery and after accidents.

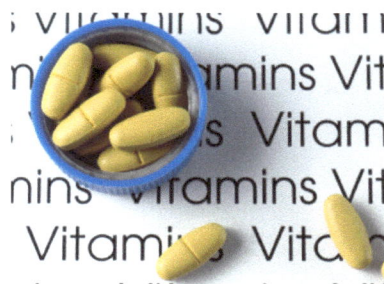

Another case study involved a Negro American who suffered severe burns to his back from a broken steam pipe. His back was a raw oozing mass of blisters that would have been extremely painful. Due to the nature of melanin which forms the dark pigment of his skin, scar tissue forms more easily. This particular burn would normally have caused severe scarring. Using a syringe, vitamin E was drawn from capsules and squirted directly onto his back. This treatment was continued daily until complete healing resulted. The rate of healing was amazing and left no scarring at all.

Cheryl Gi

VITAMIN C

Vitamin C is the most versatile and well known vitamin. It is an anti-inflammatory, antibiotic, anti-histamine, anti-toxin, anti-allergenic and much more.

- Vitamin C, also called Ascorbic Acid, is a water-soluble nutrient that is easily excreted from the body when not needed. Each of us varies greatly in our Vitamin C requirement. It's natural for one person to need 10 times as much Vitamin C as another person, and a person's age and health status can dramatically change his/her need for vitamin C.
- The amount of Vitamin C found in food varies as dramatically as our individual requirements. In general, an unripe food is much lower in Vitamin C than a ripe one, but provided that the food is ripe, the Vitamin C content is higher when the food is younger at the time of harvest.
- Vitamin C serves a predominantly protective role in the body. The protective role of Vitamin C goes far beyond our skin and gums as in the case of scurvy. Cardiovascular diseases, cancer, joint diseases and cataracts are all associated with Vitamin C deficiency and can be partly prevented by optimal intake of Vitamin C.
- Vitamin C achieves much of its protective effect by functioning as an anti-oxidant and preventing oxygen-based damage to our cells. Structures that contain fat (like the lipoprotein molecules that carry fat around our body) are particularly dependent on Vitamin C for protection.
- Poor wound healing can be a symptom of Vitamin C deficiency.
- Weak immune function, including susceptibility to colds and other infections, can also be a telltale sign of Vitamin C deficiency.
- Since the lining of our respiratory tract also depends heavily on Vitamin C for protection, respiratory infections can also be symptomatic of Vitamin C deficiency.
- In the year 2000, the National Academy of Sciences set a Tolerable Upper Intake Level (UL) for Vitamin C at

2,000 milligrams (2 grams) for adults 19 years or older. During illness a higher dose will be required. E.g. During an attack of influenza or croup.

- In my own case, I took 10,000 mg of Vitamin C daily until the worst symptoms of influenza disappeared then reduced it to 5,000 mg until recovery.
- In the U.S., one third of all adults get less Vitamin C from their diet than is recommended by the National Academy of Sciences, and 1 out of every 6 adults gets less than half the amount recommended. Smoking and exposure to second hand smoke also increase the risk of Vitamin C deficiency.
- The immune system relies on a wide variety of mechanisms to help protect the body from infection, including white blood cells, complement proteins, and interferons. *Vitamin C is especially important in the function of these immune components*.
- Vitamin C is also critical during the first phase of the body's detoxification process. This process occurs in many types of tissue, but it is especially active in the liver. When the body is exposed to toxins, Vitamin C is often required for the body to begin processing the toxins for elimination. Excessive toxic exposure increases the need for Vitamin C i.e. a higher dose is required.
- Most forms of cardiovascular disease, joint disease, cancer, eye disease, thyroid disease, liver disease, and lung disease require increased Vitamin C intake.
- Asthma, Allergies, Austism, Diabetes and all illnesses, are alleviated in some measure, with vitamin C.
- Vitamin C is required for the synthesis of collagen, an important structural component of blood vessels, tendons, ligaments, and bone.
- Vitamin C also plays an important role in the synthesis of the neurotransmitter, norepinephrine. Neurotransmitters are critical to brain function and are known to affect mood.
- In addition, Vitamin C is required for the synthesis of carnetine, which is a small molecule that is essential for the

transport of fat to cellular organelles called mitochondria, for conversion to energy.

- Recent research also suggests that Vitamin C is involved in the metabolism of cholesterol to bile acids which may have implications for blood cholesterol levels and the incidence of gallstones.

- Vitamin C is also a highly effective anti-oxidant. It can protect indispensable molecules in the body, such as proteins, lipids (fats), carbohydrates, and nucleic acids (DNA and RNA) from damage by free radicals and exposure to toxins and pollutants (e.g. smoking). Vitamin C may also be able to regenerate other anti-oxidants such as Vitamin E.

- Individuals with high blood pressure (hypertension) are at increased risk of developing cardiovascular diseases. Several studies have demonstrated a blood pressure lowering effect of Vitamin C supplementation.

- **A number of drugs are known to lower Vitamin C levels, requiring an increase in its intake: Birth control pills are known to lower vitamin C blood levels and Aspirin when taken too frequently reduces vitamin C levels by 50%.**

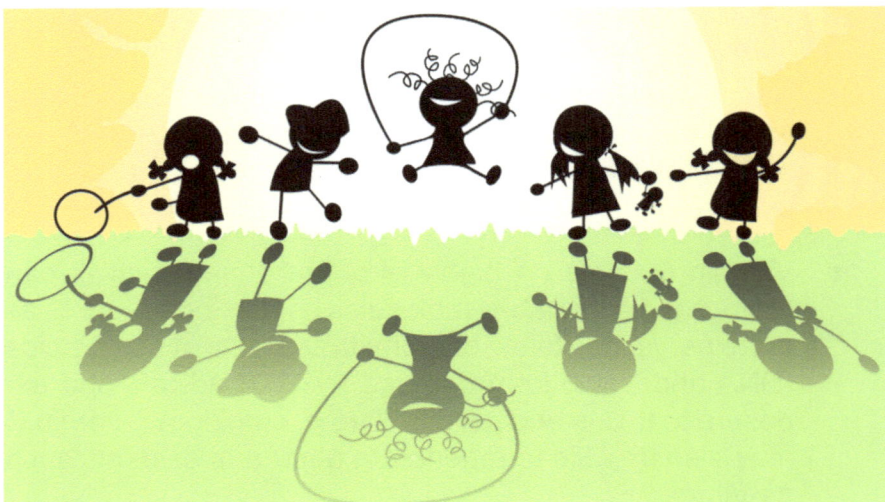

CHAPTER 9 – CAUSE AND EFFECT vs VITAMINS

The law of cause and effect operates in every area of our lives. Every situation that arises in our lives has a cause and an effect. For every choice we make or not (by default), there are consequences and for every action or lack of action there are consequences.

Do I really need to take vitamins? I have heard this argument too often.

The problem is most people base their health on how they *feel*. Just because you *feel* healthy and fit, does not mean you do not need supplements. Nor does it mean that you ARE necessarily healthy. (Refer to pages 13)

There are countless cases for example, where someone has had a cancerous growth within their body and has felt fine. The

116

late actor Michael Landon for example, was seen on a television show 3 months before he died, looking and feeling in perfect health. He was confident and convinced his health was fine, but it wasn't.

When an illness suddenly strikes, a health problem, or a sign of old age, **then** we begin to search for a supplement—**something** to help us get out of the hole we have regrettably dug ourselves into through our own inattention.

So I have to respond to the question, yes, you do need nutritional supplements.

Nutritional deficiency is almost impossible to avoid in this day and age. With our busy, fast forward lifestyle, the temptation of convenience food, it is not possible to consume the amount of nutrients our body needs. Most of the foods we eat have the nutrient value refined out of them and fresh fruit and vegetables are not what they should be anymore.

We overlook the fact that a manufacturer's primary concern is to make money. Their primary concern is NOT to promote your health. They see that as *your* responsibility.

Sixty percent (60%) of Western culture chooses to eat junk food, which is high in fat, sugar, salt and calories. It is almost devoid of any nutritional value.

Do you have recollections of the food pyramid, and just how much of each food group you have to take? I would be pretty close to the truth in saying that the majority of people haven't looked at them since high school. Unless you are one of the rare group labeled a 'health fanatic' by the general populace.

In an ideal world, health supplements should not replace the nutrients found in food. They should however complement your diet to make sure you get the full quota of nutrients that you need. Sadly, we don't live in an ideal world. Most of the fresh fruit and vegetables available no longer have the concentration of nutrients they once had.

Did you realize that you would have to eat 4 bowls of spinach today, to match the Iron from 1 bowl in 1930? This is just one example of how our soils are being depleted.

Can you imagine eating 5 kilos of wheat germ a day just to get enough Vitamin E or 5 kilos of oranges a day to get enough Vitamin C?

It isn't easy to stay away from fast foods or non-fresh foods. If your lifestyle and work conditions prevent you from having a nutritious diet, then your only hope for better health is good dietary supplements.

Just to re-cap: What are the benefits?

The most important benefit is the huge reduction in the risk of disease and the fact that you don't succumb to every 'bug' that you are exposed to. The impact of this reaches into every area of our lives with a flood of countless benefits.

There are an abundance of benefits covered extensively in the 'Answers When You Need Them' chapters, 3 to 5. Oh, and don't forget the reduced medical expenses and feeling great because you and your family are healthy, happy and in control.

Supplements help you overcome the nutritional deficiencies which contribute to ill health. We need a full range of nutrients and in full measure, for optimal health. Since our diets are not likely to provide all of them, nutritional supplements fill the gaps.

Nutritional supplements also help to boost our immune system. The stronger your immune system, the more resistant your body can be against disease – any disease.

Nutritional supplements (anti-oxidants) are also essential in getting rid of the toxins which we take in left, right and center everyday. The environmental stresses we encounter, chemicals we are exposed to, as well as our lifestyles – these all subject us to harmful toxins which undermine the utilization of nutrients and can lead to serious health problems. Anti-oxidant supplements and drinking lots of water can help our body keep toxins to a minimum.

What keeps cells from getting good nutrition?

A certain amount of the problem can be traced to the way food is grown and harvested. Chemicals, fertilizers, over-processing/ over-refining of foods- e.g. instant foods, high fat/sugar foods, foods that have been processed to make them tastier, have a longer shelf-life, etc. all contribute to extra calories. Salt and sugar can destroy vitamins and mineral.

We also keep our cells from getting good nutrition by the way we prepare our foods. We tend to over cook foods, thus taking away the minerals, vitamins and essential oils, robbing our bodies of the things that we need for proper health.

Microwaves for example, may save time but <u>they also destroy 80%</u> of the nutrient value in food. Add that to the deficiencies in our food already and we create a problem.

The toxins and free radicals that accumulate in our body every day undermine the absorption of nutrients. They both drain our nutrients and hinder assimilation. Powerful antioxidants are therefore essential.

Not drinking enough water is also a contributing factor. We overlook this basic nutrient. 90% of people are dehydrated.

Food needs to be digested, broken down into a useful micro-nutrient form and absorbed by the intestine, before any of the nutrients can be absorbed into the cells.

This means our digestive systems need to be in top condition.

The digestive system starts at the mouth all the way to the anus. If any part of the digestive system is not functioning well then assimilation of nutrients is undermined.

Have you ever tried to find out the root cause of health problems instead of running to a doctor every time you encounter minor ailments? Now you can.

Some people who take vitamins cannot see any difference. My response to that is:

They need to take a closer look at what they are taking and buying—some supplements have the amounts that would benefit a flea.

They need to be more tuned-in to the way their body functions, monitor their health, review their health history and learn to identify their body's distress signals.

Another problem is that the general populace doesn't take supplements from an informed perspective. They take the ones most available, or perhaps the cheapest or the first thing they can find in the supermarket. They assume the product is 'okay' simply because it is on the shop shelves.

Consumers believe in the advertisements from the media and the opinions of journalists. Just because the advert flashes at us like a neon sign or the newspaper headlines sensationalize an issue, doesn't mean that the claims made are genuine.

In order to ensure the integrity of a product we need to carry out our own investigations and know what to look for.

The Media who create these advertisements are another issue. The corporations and pharmaceutical companies, who make their millions out of our ill health, pay huge amounts of money for clever advertisements. They load these with psychological triggers, so that we believe what they say and keep buying.

Again, we need to do our own research instead of believing everything they say.

Take stock of your situation: If you don't notice a difference, even a subtle difference after taking supplements e.g. you are sleeping better, or you have more energy or you are more mentally alert, then try stronger supplements and make sure they are being assimilated efficiently. Perhaps enzymes are needed to assist in assimilation. To take full advantage of what dietary supplements can offer, you must choose the right supplement for you—one that gets results.

For this reason I have provided the examples of the supplements that I personally take. I have shopped around and I have certain criteria that have to be met that revolve around more value for money, high potency/quality/balance and to include a full range of nutrients. *Most importantly, they must get results— they must work.*

Having come this far with me, a person cannot plead ignorance or lack of awareness. I have taken great care to give you valuable and accurate information from health professionals to 'kick start' you on a journey towards good health. Now it's up to you.

You will be able to make an informed choice to take back control of your family's health and avoid leaving it in the hands of our struggling health system.

Remember: "If it gets the results, then it works… if it works, then it's worth pursuing"

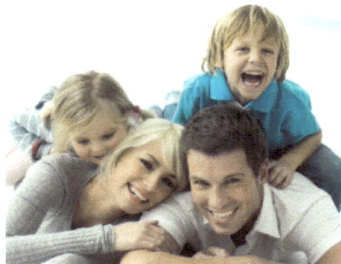

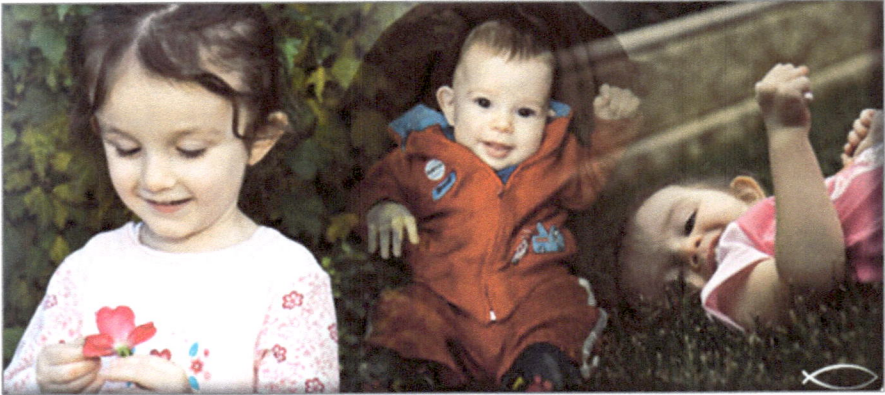

Dear Reader,

You are not alone. I will support and encourage you in your journey towards a healthy family. I wish you well.

Warmly,

Cheryl Gi

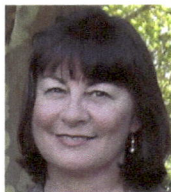

To submit questions or success stories on specific health issues,
Contact: cheryl@answers4healthykids.com

www.ingramcontent.com/pod-product-compliance
Lightning Source LLC
Chambersburg PA
CBHW060809270326
41928CB00002B/29